Anesthesiology CA-1 Pocket Survival Guide

Edited by

Mary E. Arthur, MD, FASE

Associate Professor of Anesthesiology
Department of Anesthesiology and Perioperative Medicine
Medical College of Georgia
Augusta University
Augusta, Georgia

*With Editorial Assistance by Nadine Odo
and Efrain Riveros Perez*

T0177555

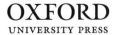

OXFORD
UNIVERSITY PRESS

OXFORD
UNIVERSITY PRESS

Oxford University Press is a department of the University of Oxford. It furthers the University's objective of excellence in research, scholarship, and education by publishing worldwide. Oxford is a registered trade mark of Oxford University Press in the UK and certain other countries.

Published in the United States of America by Oxford University Press 198 Madison Avenue, New York, NY 10016, United States of America.

© Oxford University Press 2018

CIP data is on file at the Library of Congress
ISBN 978-0-19-088588-5

This material is not intended to be, and should not be considered, a substitute for medical or other professional advice. Treatment for the conditions described in this material is highly dependent on the individual circumstances. And, while this material is designed to offer accurate information with respect to the subject matter covered and to be current as of the time it was written, research and knowledge about medical and health issues is constantly evolving and dose schedules for medications are being revised continually, with new side effects recognized and accounted for regularly. Readers must therefore always check the product information and clinical procedures with the most up- to- date published product information and data sheets provided by the manufacturers and the most recent codes of conduct and safety regulation. The publisher and the authors make no representations or warranties to readers, express or implied, as to the accuracy or completeness of this material. Without limiting the foregoing, the publisher and the authors make no representations or warranties as to the accuracy or efficacy of the drug dosages mentioned in the material. The authors and the publisher do not accept, and expressly disclaim, any responsibility for any liability, loss or risk that may be claimed or incurred as a consequence of the use and/ or application of any of the contents of this material.

9 8 7 6 5 4 3 2 1
Printed by Sheridan Books, Inc., United States of America

Contents

Contributors

Mary E. Arthur, MD, FASE
Associate Professor of Anesthesiology
Department of Anesthesiology and Perioperative Medicine
Medical College of Georgia
Augusta University
Augusta, Georgia

Vaibhav Bora, MBBS
Assistant Professor of Anesthesiology
Department of Anesthesiology and Perioperative Medicine
Medical College of Georgia
Augusta University
Augusta, Georgia

Sarah M. I. Cartwright, DNP, MSNPH, BAM, RN-BC
CAPA Integrated Clinical Practice Strategist and Adjunct Faculty
Department of Anesthesiology and Perioperative Medicine
Medical College of Georgia
Augusta University
Augusta, Georgia

Claudia F. Clavijo, MD
Assistant Professor of Anesthesiology
Department of Anesthesiology
University of Colorado Anschutz Medical Campus
Aurora, Colorado

Sanjay Dwarakanath, MD
Associate Professor of Anesthesiology
University of Kentucky
Lexington, Kentucky

Nadine Odo, CCRC, ELS
Research Associate, Medical Writer, Author's Editor
Department of Anesthesiology and Perioperative Medicine
Medical College of Georgia
Augusta University
Augusta, Georgia

Mauricio Perilla, MD
Staff Anesthesiologist and Section Head of Anesthesia
Glickman Urological Institute and Anesthesiology Institute
Cleveland Clinic
Cleveland, Ohio

Rhonda Powell, BFA
Technical Illustrator
Educational and Collaborative Technology Services
Augusta University
Augusta, Georgia

Efrain Riveros-Perez, MD
Assistant Professor of Anesthesiology
Department of Anesthesiology and Perioperative Medicine
Medical College of Georgia
Augusta University
Augusta, Georgia

CONTRIBUTORS

Lindsey Van Drunen, MD
Assistant Professor of
   Anesthesiology
University of Kentucky
Lexington, Kentucky

Ronnie Zeidan, MD
Assistant Professor of
   Anesthesiology
Department of Anesthesiology
University of Kentucky
Lexington, Kentucky

Chapter 1

What to Expect

Sanjay Dwarakanath and Lindsey Van Drunen

1.1. Orientation

The first month in anesthesiology residency can be stressful due to several factors including a new work environment, different routine, unfamiliar faces, and performance pressures, among others. An orientation is held for all specialties of incoming residents, which includes information regarding hospital-wide services. A portion of this training will likely be dedicated to technology and include an introduction to the computer system, various charting programs, and billing information. In addition, there will be an anesthesia-specific orientation. Anesthesia residency programs offer their unique version of a survival guide or orientation packet, which is a very valuable resource early on in rotations (Box 1.1). If provided, being familiar with the contents of this book can help residents jump-start their workflow and achieve competency in a *systems-based practice*.

An introductory lecture series is another way that many anesthesia programs orient their incoming residents. Didactics will be geared toward the clinical anesthesia year 1 (CA-1) residents. While these didactics will help build preliminary knowledge, they are also beneficial for the American Board of Anesthesiology (ABA) BASIC examination, which is the first in a series of staged board exams and is offered to residents at the end of their CA-1 year. Some programs also have built-in shadowing experiences with more senior residents or certified registered nurse anesthetists (CRNA). These experiences are an invaluable way to gain insight into the daily workflow of the operating room (OR), postanesthesia care unit (PACU), and/or intensive care unit (ICU). It also allows the incoming resident to gain familiarity with how to write daily progress notes or submit orders. Furthermore, shadowing experiences allow incoming residents to form relationships with already established members of the anesthesia department. These can be extremely valuable resources when CA-1 residents begin their regular anesthesia rotations and may need to "phone a friend" about management questions

Box 1.1 Important information to look for in a program's orientation book/packet

- Phone numbers, door codes
- Contact information of department personnel
- Paging system and numbers
- Lecture schedule
- Call schedules
- Rotation schedule

or even ask questions as simple as where equipment is located. Residents should take advantage of this time to ask questions and familiarize themselves with the department.

1.2. Mentor/preceptor program

Formal advising and mentoring programs are key components of an integrated professional development program in academic institutions. Residents will be assigned a faculty member who will serve as their mentor or preceptor. He or she serves as an anchorperson throughout the residency and provides a safe platform to discuss personal or professional issues at an individualized level. This is especially important to promote wellness in the workplace at a time when familiarity with department personnel is otherwise minimal. While informal meetings are available as needed, the mentor and mentee will be expected to have formal meetings every semester to ensure that key components of resident development are met (Box 1.2). In a survey done in 2016, career planning, professionalism, and achieving a balance among personal, career, and family demands seemed to be the most valuable subjects to address in a mentoring relationship.[1]

Box 1.2 Discussion items for mentors/mentees

- Personal learning goals and objectives
- Academic status and progress in the residency program
- Career plans
- Additional concerns, questions, or pertinent information

1.3. Preoperative discussion with attending the day before

As the CA-1 resident begins regular rotations in anesthesia, one of the responsibilities will be to formulate anesthetic plans for the following day's cases. At many institutions, anesthesia providers are assigned to their respective cases the day prior to when the surgery is scheduled. For example, a resident may not know the assigned cases for a Tuesday until early Monday afternoon. Once the next day's schedule is published, it is important for the resident to determine if the patients are inpatients or will be coming in from home. If admitted, inpatients may be in several different locations of the hospital such as the ICU, the floor, or the emergency department. Most academic programs expect the resident to visit the patients who are already in the hospital the day before their surgery and perform a preoperative evaluation including a physical examination. This preoperative visit serves as a learning experience and allows residents to gather missed information, identify medical issues, plan OR time efficiently, prevent last-minute delays or cancellations of the case, and, if needed, obtain further patient records from outside medical centers. An electronic medical record (EMR) is one tool to facilitate timely gathering of patient information. Most academic centers utilize an EMR, but not all hospitals use the same system. This can make record gathering time-consuming. In some instances, the patient's information may have already been synthesized, if he or she was evaluated in the preoperative anesthesia clinic. Residents should explore further information regarding the EMR and preoperative record system during the orientation period.

During the preoperative evaluation, utilization of a checklist or existing form at the local institution can help the resident perform a comprehensive evaluation and minimize missed information. This can also help organize pertinent patient details and create a good flow of conversation during presentation to the attending. Box 1.3 provides a suggested format to use for discussion with the attending. The preoperative discussion with the attending often occurs over the phone unless both the resident and attending are available in-house. Contact information for attending anesthesiologists should be provided by the institution. Consider having the pager and phone number of the assigned attending the night before the case. Investigate whether they have a preferred method of contact. Senior residents can be a good resource from which to obtain this information.

The final aspect of the preoperative discussion with the attending should include presentation of a perioperative anesthetic management plan. Organizing this plan in a systematic fashion can help the

Box 1.3 Suggested format for preoperative discussion with the attending

1. Surgical procedure and patient demographics (age, gender, and BMI)
2. Medical history by systems
3. Medications and allergies
4. Vital signs; critical care data (invasive blood pressure, central venous pressure, etc.)
5. Airway assessment; physical examination including lines; lab work
6. Tentative perioperative anesthetic management plan

resident remember to include all aspects of perioperative care. For instance, beginning with preoperative management is a good place to start. This may include epidural placement for preemptive pain control or anxiolysis. It logically progresses to intraoperative management, which can largely be broken down into three segments: induction, maintenance, and emergence from anesthesia. This section may also include planning for fluid administration, additional lines, and/or invasive monitoring. Finally, an approach to the immediate postoperative period should be presented.

1.4. Anesthesia Knowledge Test and In-Training Examination

The Anesthesia Knowledge Test (AKT) is a series of examinations that are administered at different time intervals during the residency training and are designed to assess a resident's progress. Comparisons may be made between the score obtained by one resident and those obtained by others both in his or her program and nationwide, hence providing a benchmark for individual resident assessment. Three examinations constitute the AKT: AKT-1, AKT-6, and AKT-24. The AKT-1 assesses a resident's entry-level knowledge. It is administered around the first day of residency and again at the end of the first month to determine progress made by the resident. The AKT-6 evaluates knowledge at the end of six months of training. The AKT-24 is designed to assess knowledge of a CA-2 resident whose rotations in subspecialty areas have been completed. The AKT exams are typically administered by the respective anesthesia department.

The In-Training Examination (ITE) is administered by the ABA each year to all residents enrolled in Accreditation Council for

Graduate Medical Education–accredited anesthesiology training programs, usually around the month of February during a five-day window. It will likely be proctored by support staff within the anesthesia department. The ITE is a computer-based, online exam with 200 multiple-choice questions. The purpose of this exam is to evaluate every resident's progress toward meeting the educational objectives over the continuum of education in anesthesiology. The ABA website provides complete details including the exam content and registration process. ITE scores are often expected to be reported during application for anesthesia fellowships.

1.5. Working in multidisciplinary teams

Guiding patients through the perioperative period serves as a prototypical example of the importance of working together as a team to deliver safe and effective patient care. Residents are a part of the Anesthesia Care Team (ACT), which is made up of both physicians and non-physician caregivers. Other key players in the ACT include physician anesthesiologists, CRNA, anesthesiologist assistants, and anesthesia technicians. As part of the ACT, the resident will be responsible for preoperative evaluation, prescribing the anesthetic plan, management of the anesthetic, post-anesthesia care, and anesthesia consultation. These responsibilities may span beyond the immediate pre- and postoperative periods, as anesthesiologists are becoming more widely recognized as consultant members of the perioperative surgical home. Responsibilities that may be encountered during respective perioperative periods are as follows.

Preoperative. Depending on the location of the patient encounter, the resident may have to coordinate and communicate with other teams to obtain more information or order labs or tests for preoperative optimization. Communication with the surgical team is of prime importance to understand the nature and duration of the procedure, to order relevant tests such as an echocardiogram or chest x-ray, or to request the surgical team to have an ICU bed available for an anticipated higher level of postoperative care. Communication with the nursing team often involves ordering labs (e.g., complete blood count, basic metabolic panel, or coagulation studies), administering medications (e.g., sodium citrate/citric acid commonly known as Bicitra scopolamine patch, etc.), preparing the surgical site, or ensuring completeness of paperwork such as the consent form.

Intraoperative. Close communication with the surgical team and the circulating nurse is essential during the intraoperative time. Multiple aspects of intraoperative management are often coordinated with the nursing team. Initially, this includes performing the surgical time-out, which verifies the patient's name, allergies, procedure, operative side if applicable, and antibiotic used for surgery. Furthermore, it includes sending labs as well as requesting blood products and medications. The circulating nurse also serves as an important resource for communication to other teams or areas especially when additional help is needed. Closed-loop communication with the surgical team helps members of the ACT understand the progress of the surgery, anticipate any critical events, estimate blood loss, and plan postoperative management. It is extremely important to know the channels of communication to reach the attending anesthesiologist in the event of an emergency, such as pager number, cell phone number, overhead announcement, or any other communication device that the individual hospital might have.

Postoperative. Intraoperative events often dictate the location for further transfer of care such as the ICU for critical patients or PACU followed by the hospital ward or step-down unit. Pertinent intraoperative events and a patient's medical history need to be communicated to the nursing team and the anesthesia team managing the PACU or ICU. Many institutions utilize either paper-based or computer-based hand-offs for transfer of care. This serves not only to standardize the nature of communication but also as a checklist to minimize loss of information.

Overall, the value of effective communication cannot be overlooked. It is crucial to providing the highest level of patient care, even when it takes extra effort or coordination among services. Inevitably, the role of anesthesiologist as consultant will continue to grow. It is more important now than ever before to remember that if anesthesia professionals are not involved and not perceived as interested, dedicated team players, they will be shut out of critical negotiations and decisions relevant to their practice.

Further Reading

American Board of Anesthesiology. In-training examination blueprint. http://www.theaba.org/PDFs/ITE-Exam/ITE-Exam-Blueprint. Accessed January 16, 2018.

Correll DJ, Bader AM, Hull MW, Hsu C, Tsen LC, Hepner DL. Value of preoperative clinic visits in identifying issues with potential impact on operating room efficiency. *Anesthesiology.* 2006;105(6):1254–1259.

Eichhorn JH, Grider JS. Scope of practice. In: Barash PG. et al., eds. *Clinical Anesthesia,* 7th ed. Philadelphia, PA: Lippincott Williams & Wilkins; 2013:32–36.

Gonzalez LS, ML. A survey of residency program directors in anesthesiology. *J Clin Anesth.* 2016;33:254–265.

Chapter 2

Making the Most of Your CA-1 Year

Mary E. Arthur and Vaibhav Bora

Introduction

Making the transition from the clinical base year to the first clinical anesthesia year (CA-1) can be stressful as residents continue their journey toward independent practice. Adhering to a few simple rules can smooth that journey considerably.

2.1. Do's and Don'ts

Be prepared. Orientation will cover institutional and departmental policies, procedures, structure, and operation. During orientation, an overview will be given of Accreditation Council for Graduate Medical Education (ACGME) requirements, the department's specific program requirements, and American Board of Anesthesiology (ABA) eligibility criteria for the ABA BASIC examination. The orientation period is a good time to create online accounts, including an ACGME account to be able to enter case logs, an institutional account to record duty hours and evaluations, and an ABA account to register for the BASIC exam and receive ABA updates.

Set up the operating room: Residents should come in early to set up the room. A thorough anesthesia setup includes machine checkout; a functional suction system; drawing up medications for the case and labeling syringes with medication name, concentration, date, and time the medications were drawn; and set up of airway equipment, intravenous kits, and any special equipment that may be needed.

Introduce yourself to the nurses and ancillary staff in the room These health care professionals will help you, welcome you, and make you feel comfortable in the room. Because of rapid physiologic responses of the patient, unforeseen surgical events, and external influences such as time pressures for the efficient use of the operating room, teamwork is essential for team performance, patient safety, and good outcomes in anesthesia and perioperative care. Different professional groups with conflicting needs and priorities with differing interpersonal relationships work closely together to ensure patient safety while maintaining efficient work flow.

Always do a thorough preoperative evaluation with a good airway assessment the day prior to your case for inpatients. If your patient is admitted on the morning of surgery, give yourself enough time to meet the patient in the holding area and go over the history and physical exam. This will give you an opportunity to reevaluate the airway and formulate an anesthetic plan.

Read up on your cases the day before. Good resources are the textbooks *Basics of Anesthesia* by Miller and *Clinical Anesthesiology* by Morgan and Mikhail.

Call the attending assigned to your case the night before to discuss the patient's relevant information and an anesthetic plan. Always read up and have a basic understanding of the procedure, know your patient, and have an anesthetic plan before calling.

Call your attending if you need help. Do not attempt to troubleshoot problems by yourself, especially during the early stages of training. You are there to learn, and your attending and senior residents are there to help you.

Do not leave the patient unattended: Beginning CA-1 residents have been known to step out of the operating room when they thought the patient was stable to pick up necessary medications or equipment. This is unacceptable. According to ASA standards for basic anesthetic monitoring, STANDARD 1, qualified anesthesia personnel shall be present in the room throughout the conduct of all general anesthetics, regional anesthetics, and monitored anesthesia care.

Patients should be attended to *at all times*. If there is a need, the attending should be paged, or an anesthesia tech or another available resident should be asked to pick up what is needed.

Do not make major decisions without consulting your attending relating to

- Blood transfusion
- Electrolyte replacement, especially potassium
- Procedures—require attending's authorization and supervision
- Extubation—requires consultation with attending
- Crucial or difficult conversations with the surgical/nursing team or with the patient or family

Refer to Figure 2.1.

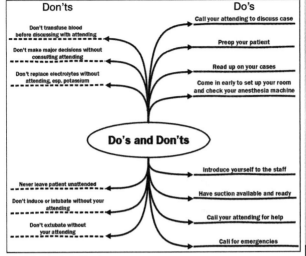

Don'ts	Do's
Don't transfuse blood before discussing with attending	Call your attending to discuss case
Don't make major decisions without consulting attending	Preop your patient
Don't replace electrolytes without attending, esp. potassium	Read up on your cases
	Come in early to set up your room and check your anesthesia machine

Do's and Don'ts

Don'ts	Do's
Never leave patient unattended	Introduce yourself to the staff
Don't induce or intubate without your attending	Have suction available and ready
Don't extubate without your attending	Call your attending for help
	Call for emergencies

Figure 2.1. Do's and Don'ts

2.2. Speak Up

In 2002, the Joint Commission launched the Speak Up patient safety program. Over time, the program, which encourages patients to speak up and be active participants in their health care, has expanded to more than 70 countries. Under the same concept, it is important that, during the transition from internship to clinical anesthesia, CA-1 residents speak up and be active participants in their training and education. Appreciating assertive behavior will further improve team performance (Figure 2.2).

Speak up with any questions or concerns. Attendings and senior residents understand how stressful the first few months can be for those new to the specialty. It is important to ask questions and get clarifications; you will not be faulted for it.

Pay attention to detail and the care you give. As someone new to the specialty, give yourself enough time to prepare by arriving early to set up your room, go over your preoperative note, meet your patient, and evaluate the patient's airway.

Educate yourself about the patient's comorbidities and the surgical procedure. Understanding the procedure and knowing your patient's medical history, including drugs the patient is on and has taken on the morning of surgery, will help you deliver a good anesthetic and take good care of your patient.

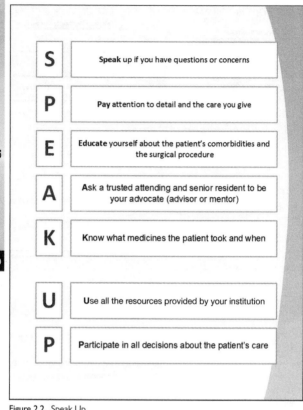

S	**Speak** up if you have questions or concerns
P	**Pay** attention to detail and the care you give
E	**Educate** yourself about the patient's comorbidities and the surgical procedure
A	**Ask** a trusted attending and senior resident to be your advocate (advisor or mentor)
K	**Know** what medicines the patient took and when
U	**Use** all the resources provided by your institution
P	**Participate** in all decisions about the patient's care

Figure 2.2. Speak Up

Ask a trusted attending and senior resident to be your advocate (advisor or mentor). All residency programs have mentorship programs in place in which incoming CA-1 residents are assigned to a faculty mentor and sometimes a senior resident for guidance. The programs also give residents time to familiarize themselves with the department staff to find a faculty member of their choice with whom they can relate and work well. Feel free to approach your program director if you are not assigned a mentor.

Know the patient's medication history as it may influence the anesthetic management. For instance, patients on angiotensin receptor blockers who take their medications on the morning of surgery may have intractable hypotension after induction of anesthesia. Having this knowledge will help you have drugs ready to treat any intraoperative hypotension.

Use all the resources provided by your institution to maximize your educational experience. Some programs provide online question banks (e.g., TrueLearn) or online resources (e.g., Anesthesia Toolbox) that can be accessed remotely and have interactive modules. Anesthesia Toolbox is an online learning management system with various resources including lectures and podcasts which have undergone rigorous peer review. Experts from different anesthesia programs and subspecialties have contributed to these websites to ensure that information is uniform across anesthesia residencies in the United States (https://www.anesthesiatoolbox.com/).

Participate in all decisions related to patient care.

2.3. Professionalism

Professionalism starts with a commitment and devotion to quality, excellence, and personal sacrifice that goes beyond an eight-hour day. It must rest on a solid base of education, experience, and skill and must encompass real respect for other professionals as well as patients.

Professionalism forms the core of all we do to become good anesthesiologists. It is central to our commitment to our patients, medical institutions, departments, communities, and colleagues.

The principal aim of graduate medical education is to prepare doctors for safe independent practice of medicine and also expose residents to the demands of real-life practice, including the long work hours on completion of residency or fellowship.

The professional responsibilities of an anesthesiology resident include

- Appearing for duty appropriately rested and fit to provide the services required by your patients
- The ability to demonstrate an understanding and acceptance of your personal role in assuring the safety and welfare of patients entrusted to your care
- The provision of patient and family-centered care
- Time management before, during, and after clinical assignments
- The recognition of impairment including illness and fatigue in yourself and your peers
- A commitment to lifelong learning
- Monitoring your patient care performance and being accountable for improvement indicators
- Accurately and honestly reporting duty hours, patient outcomes, and clinical experience data
- Appearing at work professionally dressed

A neat, clean appearance is desired by patients even in this era of more casual attire. Scrub suits should be clean and unstained, and, outside the operating room, a clean white coat over the scrub suit is essential.

Residents should take ownership of their patients and always remember to conduct themselves as physicians concerned for the patient's well-being. A resident's responsibilities are not over once the airway is secured. Residents should empathically listen to patient's concerns, explain the therapeutic options honestly and openly, and recommend an anesthetic plan. Equally important is the need to acknowledge autonomy in determining the treatment plan. By practicing in an honest and compassionate manner, we fulfill our obligations as medical professionals.

2.4. Interpersonal and communication skills

Interpersonal and communication skills are among the core competencies of the ACGME. To achieve these milestones, residents must demonstrate skills to effectively exchange information and collaborate with patients, their families, and other members of the health care team while being empathic. Residents should be able to communicate effectively with faculty, their peers, surgeons, other members of the health care team, and health-related agencies. They should be able to act in the role of a consultant and be able to discuss information with patients from a broad range of socioeconomic and cultural backgrounds. Maintaining comprehensive, timely, and legible medical records is also required. Preoperatively, residents are required to review the patient medical history, history of past anesthetics, allergies, and medications and communicate this information effectively to the attending anesthesiologist and other members of the health care team.

SBAR, an acronym for Situation, Background, Assessment, Recommendation, is a powerful tool that is used to improve the effectiveness of communication between individuals. It is easy to implement and can help residents learn the key components needed to send a complete message (Figure 2.3).

SBAR can be used when signing out to the postanesthesia care unit (PACU) nurses or the intensive care unit (ICU) staff and in the context of perioperative consultation. Intraoperatively, residents should participate in "time out" as well as other patient safety protocols, using the Speak Up strategy, and bring issues that may

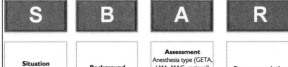

Figure 2.3. SBAR

affect patient safety to the attention of the team. Postoperatively, residents should communicate all relevant information to the PACU/ICU team and provide medical guidance. Effective communication improves patient satisfaction, minimizes error in patient care, helps to build collegial relations with physicians and providers from other specialties, and can protect from litigation.

2.5. Work-life balance

Anesthesiology residents make life and death decisions every day, often in very difficult emergency situations and during long shifts. Residents may feel a personal responsibility for an intraoperative death. The resulting stress can take its toll over time, resulting in difficulty sleeping, lack of appetite, clinical depression, and other serious issues. Female residents have specific gender-related stressors. They have to reconcile multiple roles, such as balancing career, relationships, child bearing, and child rearing. In addition, certain biological factors may make residents vulnerable to mood disturbances (Table 2.1).

Table 2.1. Biological factors may make residents more vulnerable to mood disturbances	
1.	Lack of sleep
2.	Poor eating habits
3.	Poor level of fitness
4.	A positive family history of mental illness
5.	Physical illness

Residents may be vulnerable to substance abuse because of these stressors. Anesthesiology residents represent 4.6% of the US resident population but constitute 33.7% of all residents in the Medical Association of Georgia's Impaired Physician Program. The incidence of substance abuse in anesthesiology residencies has remained steady at 1% to 2% despite the increased numbers of hours of education incorporated into residency training. Returning to anesthesiology residency after a substance-related absence has a high failure rate (50%), and the risk of relapse can be lethal, with an alarmingly high incidence of suicide or lethal overdose.

Once the work-life balance is tilted in the favor of work, residents become overwhelmed, and burnout sets in. It is important not to allow work to be overwhelming. The ASA and ACGME have placed a huge emphasis on resident wellness, and there are several institutional and departmental resources that can help.

2.6. Burnout and reaching out

Anesthesiology residency is challenging physically, psychologically, and intellectually. Because of the skills and concepts required in an environment that requires rapid decision-making, trainees may experience uncertainty in their knowledge and clinical abilities. Burnout is a psychological syndrome of emotional exhaustion, depersonalization, and reduced personal accomplishment, and it can lead to a decline in both quantity and quality of medical care. It is characterized by personal dissatisfaction as well as poor and uninspired work performance. It represents a deterioration of values, dignity, and spirit that spreads gradually and continuously over time, sending physicians into a depressive downward spiral from which it is hard to recover. The risk of burnout increases in individuals who consistently experience work overload and perceive a lack of control over the extent to which work duties exceed their capacity. Individuals affected by burnout withdraw emotionally from colleagues and patients, become apathetic and sad, and think of work only as a means of earning a living. They lose interest, enthusiasm, and motivation to do their best for their patients. Inevitably their personal life suffers as well.

Chronic overstress is described as burnout. Initially, the individual feels emotionally exhausted but is still able to get through the day at work, with little else to give. Afterwards, the person is exhausted, irritable, and impatient. It becomes so difficult to be with others that social withdrawal, depersonalization, and isolation become evident. The affected resident begins to feel negative about people and work that used to be enjoyable, and then develops a reduced sense of accomplishment and satisfaction from work to the point of becoming cynical and distant. Physicians at this stage often consider leaving the profession.

The five early signs of burnout, which may be precursors to depression, are listed in Table 2.2.

Performance errors, which can result from physical and emotional exhaustion, cynicism, and depersonalization, can in turn lead to more burnout and distress. Recent reports have also revealed an increase in drug errors made by depressed residents.

As a beginning CA-1 resident, what can you do to prevent burnout? First, focus on what you can control. The best approach to dealing with stress is to identify the cause of the stress and what part of it is under your control, then focus on that.

A suggested approach for dealing with stress is as follows.

Take care of yourself: Make time for yourself, eat regular healthy meals daily, exercise regularly and stay fit, learn relaxation techniques, and develop good sleep habits. Every beginning CA-1 resident should have a family doctor and keep up with yearly visits. It is important to manage your time efficiently at work by being organized, keeping realistic schedules, and not overcommitting yourself. Recognizing and accepting that you cannot do everything; setting priorities that include yourself, your family, and friends; setting and maintaining limits; and learning to say "no" while realizing that trying to please everyone is not in your best interest is key to a successful transition into residency.

Take regular breaks and vacations. Do not wait for a crisis. Do something you want to do, not something you have to do.

Anticipate and prepare for situations, both at home and work. Set realistic expectations of yourself.

Make it a rule not to take your work home. If you do, it should be the rare exception to the rule. Give your family your full attention when you are with them.

Laugh more often. Look for and enjoy humor on a regular basis. Share a laugh with family, friends, and colleagues. Add fun to work.

Table 2.2. Early signs of burnout	
1	An increase in physical problems and illnesses
2	Escalating problems with relationships
3	An enhanced frequency of negative thoughts and feelings
4	A significant increase in unhealthy habits, such as overeating, not exercising, smoking, an increase in alcohol or drug intake, or lateness at work
5	Fatigue or exhaustion

Have at least one good friend. Share concerns with trusted colleagues. Reach out and get a mentor. Ask for help if needed. Foster team spirit at work.

Make your family a priority. Take time for yourself and your family without feeling guilt.

Create a financial plan. Stick to the basic principles, reduce nondeductible debts, and plan to save. Do not live beyond your means. Being financially overcommitted is the second most common reason that physicians do not make changes to decrease their level of stress. While the stress of residency will always be present, we can work to keep it positive, motivating, and enriching.

2.7. Examinations

Certification in anesthesiology is an objective way of assessing a physician's progress in his or her career. The ABA is the certifying body for anesthesiologists. This nonprofit organization is a member board of the American Board of Medical Specialties. The board administers primary and subspecialty certification exams as well as the Maintenance of Certification in Anesthesiology (MOCA) program, which aims at promoting lifelong learning and ensuring quality of care and patient safety.

2.7.1. Anesthesia Knowledge Tests

Some programs administer the Anesthesia Knowledge Test (AKT) series to determine the extent to which a resident has progressed in knowledge. The series includes three examinations: the AKT-1 administered during the first month of residency, the AKT-6 administered during the sixth month of residency, and the AKT-24 administered during the 24th month of residency. Some programs also assess entering residents' knowledge by allowing them to take the AKT-1 on the first day of the CA-1 year as a pre-AKT and the post-AKT-1 30 days after starting the CA-1 year.

2.7.2. In-Training Exam

The In-Training Exam (ITE) is administered every year to all anesthesiology residents. It is a four-hour computer-based exam consisting of 200 multiple-choice questions. Each residency program administers the exam at its site. The ITE is a formative examination designed to evaluate a resident's progress toward meeting the educational objectives of the continuum of education in anesthesiology. Programs monitor resident progress by performance on the ITE, and each institution comes out with its ITE pass rate. In general a scaled score of 30 and above on the ITE correlates with a BASIC exam pass rate of greater than 96%.

The ITE covers both basic and advanced topics in four content categories:

- Basic sciences
- Clinical sciences
- Organ-based basic and clinical sciences
- Special problems or issues in anesthesiology

Table 2.3 shows the number and relative percentage of questions from each of the four content categories.

2.7.3. BASIC Exam

CA-1 residents can only advance in their training after successfully passing the ABA BASIC examination. The staged examinations (i.e., the BASIC and Advanced examinations) complement ACGME competency-based training and promotion.

The BASIC examination, the first exam in the series, is offered to residents at the end of their CA-1 year. It focuses on the scientific basis of clinical anesthetic practice and concentrates on content areas such as pharmacology, physiology, anatomy, anesthesia equipment, and monitoring. The ABA website provides content outline which helps in preparation for the test (http://www.theaba.org/PDFs/BASIC-Exam/Basic-and-Advanced-ContentOutline). The ABA website also provides policies and procedures, and residents are strongly encouraged to read these when preparing for their boards (http://www.theaba.org/PDFs/

Table 2.3. ITE blueprint

Basic topics in anesthesiology (50%)		Advanced topics in anesthesiology (50%)	
Content	Number of questions	Content	Number of questions
Basic sciences (12%)	21–29	Basic sciences (4%)	6–10
Clinical sciences (17%)	29–43	Clinical sciences (4%)	6–10
Organ-based basic and clinical sciences (19%)	30–46	Organ-based basic and clinical sciences (15%)	22–38
Special problems or issues in anesthesiology (2%)	2–6	Special problems or issues in anesthesiology (3%)	6–14
		Clinical subspecialties (24%)	36–60

Table 2.4. Basic blueprint	
Content category (relative percentage)	Number of questions
Basic sciences (24%)	44–52
Clinical sciences (36%)	65–79
Organ-based basic and clinical sciences (37%)	66–82
Special problems or issues in anesthesiology (3%)	4–8

BOI/StagedExaminations-BOI). The questions are single correct answer type multiple-choice questions, and sample questions can be found on the ABA website (http://www.theaba.org/PDFs/BASIC-Exam/BASIC-Sample-Questions).

Start preparing for the exam early. An ABA blueprint showing the distribution of questions is available on the ABA website (http://www.theaba.org/PDFs/BASIC-Exam/BASIC-Exam-Blueprint). The content is broadly divided into the same categories as the ITE. Table 2.4 shows the number and relative percentage of questions from each of the four content categories.

The BASIC examination consists of 200 questions, and examinees have four hours to complete it. The BASIC includes A-type items only. A-type questions are single best answer multiple-choice questions that require the application of knowledge rather than simple recall of factual information. These questions often include a brief clinical vignette followed by a lead-in question and four response options. Some questions reference static images.

The ABA has also provided a sample timeline for staged exams (Figure 2.4). It is important for CA-1 residents to familiarize themselves with the timeline in order to apply for the test and prepare themselves for taking it in a timely manner.

2.7.4. Registration eligibility and dates

To register for the BASIC examination, the clinical competency committee of the training program must certify the resident as having satisfactorily completed *18 months* of training. This includes 12 months of clinical base training (internship) and 6 months of clinical anesthesiology training.

Residents should complete this requirement before March 31 of a particular year to be eligible to register for the summer BASIC examination. Residents who complete this requirement before *September 30* of the same year may register for the fall BASIC examination.

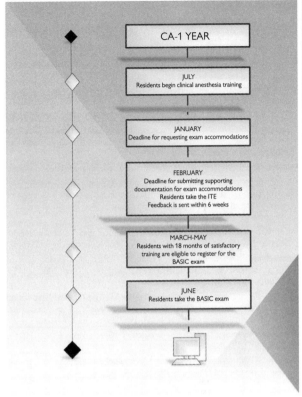

Figure 2.4. Timeline for BASIC Exam

2.7.5. Maintenance of certification in anesthesiology program

Learning does not end with certification. The MOCA 2.0 program provides diplomates with opportunities to continuously learn and demonstrate proficiencies in providing better patient care by offering a relevant and personalized approach to helping diplomates to assess their knowledge and address knowledge gaps.

Start early in your CA-1 year, because this will be a lifelong endeavor to continuously learn and improve.

Further Reading

Butterworth JF, Mackey DC, Wasnick JD. *Morgan & Mikhail's Clinical Anesthesiology*. New York: McGraw-Hill; 2013.

Fahrenkopf AM, Sectish TC, Barger LK, et al. Rates of medication errors among depressed and burnt out residents: prospective cohort study. *BMJ*. 2008;336(7642):488–491.

Gautam, M. Before burnout: how physicians can defuse stress. *The virtual mentor: VM*. 2003;5(9):61–66.

Silverman MM. Physicians and suicide. In: Goldman LS, Myers M, Dickstein LJ, eds. *The Handbook of Physician Health: The Essential Guide to Understanding the Health Care Needs of Physicians*. Chicago: American Medical Association; 2000: 95–117.

Maslach C, Leiter MP. *The Truth about Burnout*. San Francisco: Jossey-Bass; 1997.

Menk EJ, Baumgarten RK, Kingsley CP, Culling RD, Middaugh R. Success of reentry into anesthesiology training programs by residents with a history of substance abuse. *JAMA*. 1990;263(22):3060–3062.

Miller RD, Pardo M. *Basics of Anesthesia*. Philadelphia: Elsevier Health Sciences; 2011.

Schartel SA, Kuhn C, Culley DJ, Wood M, Cohen N. Development of the anesthesiology educational milestones. *J Grad Med Educ*. 2014;6 (1 Suppl. 1):12–14.

Talbott GD, Gallegos KV, Wilson PO, Porter TL. The Medical Association of Georgia's Impaired Physicians Program: review of the first 1000 physicians: analysis of specialty. *JAMA*. 1987;257(21):2927–2930.

The anesthesiology milestone project. *J Grad Med Educ*. 2014;6 (1 Suppl. 1):15–28.

Williams GW, Williams ES. *Basic Anesthesiology Examination Review*. New York: Oxford University Press; 2016.

Chapter 3

Preanesthesia Patient Evaluation

Efrain Riveros-Perez and Mauricio Perilla

Introduction

A thorough preanesthesia medical evaluation includes a review of pertinent medical records, an interrogation of the patient, and a focused physical exam. This evaluation triggers additional diagnostic tests and consultations and serves as a foundation to devise an anesthetic plan.

3.1. Preadmission testing

3.1.1. Evaluating the patient

3.1.1.1. Preanesthesia screening

The approach to the preanesthesia evaluation must be comprehensive, accurate, and efficient. The use of resources—personnel, time, and infrastructure—should be based on the expected benefits in the context of system efficiency. With the growth of ambulatory procedures and same-day admissions, medical institutions have begun to implement preanesthesia screening systems to identify high-risk patients, avoid unnecessary testing, and minimize delays, postponements, and cancellations, thereby improving patient satisfaction and quality of care.

The system can be implemented via telephone contact or in an interactive online modality. Preanesthesia screening should ideally use web-based technologies, quality improvement techniques, and patient-centered services. An interactive website which allows patients to fill out their own medical history at a time convenient to them makes it easy for them to provide the necessary information. The web-based system can also be used to educate patients about their upcoming procedure and discharge process. Conducting preanesthesia screening by phone is associated with staffing costs, especially as it can be difficult for the nurse and patient to connect, creating a phone tag situation. With the online system, on the other hand, the questionnaire is often not fully completed. In any case, combining both modalities, with phone calls arranged for patients unable or unwilling to access the online system, might produce more complete coverage of the scheduled patients. A structured questionnaire with screening health-related questions (Table 3.1) and an algorithm-driven standard anesthesia guideline (Figure 3.1) identify high-risk patients and cases that require additional work-up and consultations.

3.1.1.2. Physical status and comorbidities

The goal of the preanesthesia evaluation is to assess the patient's medical condition and ability to tolerate the physiologic changes associated with anesthesia and surgery in order to develop an anesthetic plan that expedites recovery and patient satisfaction. A comprehensive evaluation should include

- Present illness—indication for surgery and physiologic effects of surgical condition.
- Medical history—diagnosed medical problems involving different organ systems (i.e., cardiovascular, respiratory, neurologic, gastrointestinal, metabolic, hematologic, and musculoskeletal).
- Allergies—latex, tape, and medications.

Table 3.1. Sample preanesthesia screening questionnaire

	Do you?	Yes	No
1	Have a history of cardiac problems (heart attack, chest pain, heart surgery, cardiac stents, or irregular heart beat?	☐	☐
2	Have a history of stroke or brain aneurysm?	☐	☐
3	Have breathing problems or history of COPD, asthma, sleep apnea, or use oxygen or CPAP machine at home?	☐	☐
4	Have a pacemaker or defibrillator?	☐	☐
5	Have kidney problems requiring any type of dialysis?	☐	☐
6	Take blood thinners other than aspirin (Plavix, Coumadin, Eliquis, Pradaxa) for any reason?	☐	☐
8	Have diabetes and use insulin?	☐	☐
9	Get chest pain or shortness of breath after climbing a flight stairs?	☐	☐

If the patient answers yes to any of the above questions, please schedule an office appointment with the anesthesiologist.

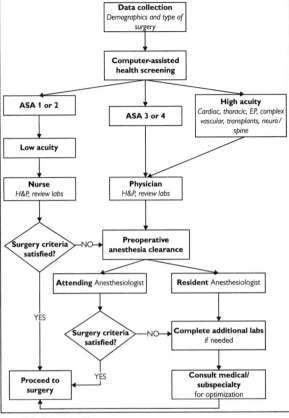

Figure 3.1. Triage algorithm

- Past anesthetic history—intra- and postoperative complications, history of difficult airway, metabolic disturbances (e.g., atypical pseudocholinesterase, malignant hyperthermia), and postoperative nausea and vomiting.
- Family history—genetic disorders with anesthetic implications, adverse reactions to anesthesia.
- Functional class.
- Review of systems—symptoms related to organ systems.
- Physical exam—airway examination, cardiopulmonary evaluation, and general physical assessment.

- Interpretation of laboratory and imaging tests as well as consultation reports.
- Determination of physical status.
- Anesthetic plan and informed consent discussion.

The American Society of Anesthesiologists (ASA) physical status classification is routinely used to assess the patient's overall health status. While this tool is not intended to stratify risks, the classes are associated with risk of mortality, length of stay, costs, unexpected admissions, and postoperative intensive care admissions (Table 3.2).

The effect of different comorbidities on the clinical status of the patient should be optimized to mitigate the risk associated with them. This optimization may require additional consultations and tests as well as the use of medications. For instance, bronchospasm in a patient with severe chronic obstructive pulmonary disease would typically be addressed with preoperative respiratory treatments and bronchodilator therapy. Depending on the case, a pulmonology consultation and pulmonary function tests may be indicated.

3.1.1.3. Medication reconciliation

Medication reconciliation—the process of comparing the medications that the patient is taking with the list of ordered medications—is a major component of safe care. Since admission of a surgical patient represents a transition of care, the preanesthesia setting is ideal for this process to avoid order duplication, dosing errors, omissions, and drug interactions. Recommendations for medications to be taken the day before and the day of surgery should be made at this time.

3.1.1.4. Risk stratification

The assessment of overall patient risk must include the risks related to the patient's clinical status and those associated with

Table 3.2. ASA physical status classification	
ASA I	A normal healthy patient
ASA II	189.15 pt
ASA III	A patient with severe systemic disease
ASA IV	A patient with severe systemic disease that is a constant threat to life
ASA V	A moribund patient who is not expected to survive without the operation
ASA VI	A declared brain dead patient whose organs are being removed for transplant

> ## Box 3.1 RCRI risk factors
>
> - Ischemic heart disease
> - Heart failure
> - Cerebrovascular disease
> - Diabetes mellitus requiring insulin
> - Serum creatinine ≥2.0 mg/dL
> - High-risk surgery (intraperitoneal, intrathoracic, or suprainguinal vascular procedures)
>
> Adapted from Lee TH, Marcantonio ER, Mangione CM, et al. Derivation and prospective validation of a simple index for prediction of cardiac risk of major non cardiac surgery. *Circulation*. 1999;100:1043.

the surgical intervention. In addition to ASA physical status and functional class, complex scoring systems have been developed to stratify patients and predict perioperative risk (Box 3.1). These multifactorial scoring systems are available as easy-to-use calculators to quantify overall risk. The most commonly used risk stratification systems are the Revised Cardiac Risk Index (RCRI) and the National Surgical Quality Improvement Program (NSQIP) risk calculator (Box 3.2).

The risk stratification systems allow the practitioner to anticipate perioperative complications and to plan for implementation of specific monitoring strategies and therapies as well as postoperative

> ## Box 3.2 Parameters evaluated by the NSQIP risk calculator
>
> - Planned procedure
> - Gender
> - Functional status
> - Emergency case
> - ASA physical status
> - Steroid use for chronic condition
> - Ascites within 30 days prior to surgery
> - Diabetes
> - Hypertension requiring medication
> - Congestive heart failure within 30 days prior to surgery
> - Dyspnea
> - Current smoker within one year
> - History of severe COPD
> - Dialysis

disposition. It is of paramount importance to discuss risks with the patient as part of the informed consent process.

3.1.1.5. Preoperative testing

Preoperative laboratory testing should be ordered based on information gathered during the preanesthesia evaluation. Testing should be used to modify a pretest probability established on clinical assessment rather than to diagnose a "hidden" condition without clinical risk or manifestations. In the absence of clinical indications, laboratory testing is not recommended, given the low predictive value of an abnormal test in a healthy population with low prevalence for a disease. The same holds true for other diagnostic exams such as electrocardiogram, echocardiogram, and pulmonary function tests.

While routine preoperative testing is not generally indicated, in some instances selective testing might be useful in high-risk specific surgical procedures. The following tests should be considered:

- Hemoglobin and hematocrit—baseline level for procedures with significant anticipated blood loss.
- Platelet count—baseline level when neuraxial blocks are considered during pregnancy.
- Pregnancy test—although controversial, it is reasonable in childbearing-age patients as long as the result affects the surgical or anesthetic plan.

3.1.1.6. Informed consent

Active patient participation in the decision-making process is desirable throughout the perioperative journey. Discussing the anesthetic plan and its benefits, complications, alternatives, and risks facilitates communication between the patient and the care team while improving patient satisfaction and reducing anxiety. The informed consent should be conceived as a process rather than as documentation signing. Once the anesthesia care provider gathers all the required information and devises an anesthetic plan, it should be presented in a systematic and easy-to-understand fashion to facilitate shared decisions with the patient, creating an environment of trust in which all questions can be addressed appropriately. An anesthesia resident who is obtaining the consent should identify him or herself and his or her role and reassure the patient that the attending anesthesiologist agrees with the plan.

Several aspects of the informed consent deserve mention. Although anesthetic procedures occur simultaneously with surgical interventions, the nuances of anesthetic procedures warrant specific discussion beyond the broad surgical consent. Consent to receive transfusion of blood products must be obtained as part of the anesthesia discussion; when a patient refuses transfusions, consent to individual blood product fractions must be addressed and the consent must reflect the patient's wishes. Do not resuscitate orders should be addressed with the patient, family members, and surrogates in order to clarify specific levels of resuscitation (pharmacologic support, tracheal intubation, defibrillation). The results of that discussion as well as instructions for order reinstatement should be appropriately documented.

3.1.1.7. Patient instructions

After a thorough discussion of the anesthetic plan with the patient, specific instructions regarding what to expect on the day of surgery and where to check in should be provided. Patient education is paramount and should include preoperative fasting guidelines and the use of preoperative medications. In addition to verbal explanations, booklets and online resources are advised to facilitate compliance. Finally, the preanesthesia visit is an excellent opportunity to provide counsel in general health issues such as smoking cessation and healthy habits (Table 3.3).

3.1.1.8. Documentation of evaluation

The anesthesia provider is responsible for accurately documenting the results and analysis from the preanesthesia evaluation. This information is helpful for the anesthesiologist assigned to the case on the day of surgery. The documentation must include

- Patient identification
- Identification of surgical procedure
- Allergies
- Functional class
- Relevant medical history
  - Medical history
  - Anesthesia history
  - Family history
- Physical examination
  - Vital signs, weight, and body mass index
  - Airway exam

Table 3.3. Preoperative fasting recommendations	
Clear liquids	2 hours
Breast milk	4 hours
Non-human milk	6 hours
Light meal	6 hours
Heavy meal	8 hours

- Cardiopulmonary exam
- General physical exam
- Relevant laboratory testing and imaging results
- Relevant consultation reports
- Assignment of ASA physical status and case analysis
- Anesthesia plan
  - Preoperative recommendations and premedication
  - Intraoperative plan and monitoring
  - Postoperative disposition
- Informed consent and counseling
- Presence of advance directives

3.1.2. Communicating the evaluation

Anesthesia residents are expected to summarize the preanesthesia evaluation in a logical and comprehensive fashion to convey the relevant information to other team members. Feedback after communicating with the primary surgical service is of particular importance either to clear the patient for surgery or to notify the primary service that additional testing and/or consultations are necessary. Adequate coordination between anesthesiologists and surgeons is critical to ensure safe care, optimize case scheduling, and improve patient satisfaction. The anesthesia resident must discuss the case with the anesthesiologist in charge of the preanesthesia clinic and in special circumstances also with the anesthesiologist assigned to perform the anesthetic the day of surgery. Communication between resident and the anesthesia attending should take place before the final recommendations are given to the patient. Under no circumstances should the resident see a patient alone before the scheduling process continues.

3.2. Preanesthesia evaluation in special circumstances

Although a significant proportion of surgical patients are admitted the day of surgery, inpatients frequently require surgical interventions. Additionally, some special situations require attention to unique aspects of the case and include patients in the acute care setting, obstetric patients, and patients with cardiac morbidities scheduled for noncardiac operations.

3.2.1. Acute care settings

Early involvement of the anesthesiology service in the evaluation of patients in the acute care setting including trauma is critical, as an interdisciplinary approach is associated with better outcomes. The acutely ill patient has alterations at different organ levels. The initial evaluation should be focused on specific aspects including preoperative fasting status, degree of hemodynamic and respiratory compromise, airway assessment, and metabolic derangements. A systematic and organized approach is useful to rapidly diagnose life-threatening conditions and treat them before taking the patient to the operating room.

Anesthesia in the trauma setting is particularly challenging. Preanesthesia evaluation in such cases consists of an initial primary survey to identify life-threatening conditions and potential neurologic injury followed by a secondary survey to examine the patient from head to toe. As part of the secondary evaluation, the anesthesiologist must assess the airway and the progression of both the cardiovascular and pulmonary condition. Constant communication with the surgical team and nursing staff plays a pivotal role in the initial evaluation and management of the patient in the emergency room and during transfer to the operating room. The clinical condition of the trauma patient might change in a short period, warranting constant attention to these dynamic changes by the anesthesiologist to adjust the anesthetic plan accordingly.

3.2.2. Obstetrics

The physiologic changes of pregnancy involve almost every organ system. The anesthesiologist must be aware of these changes and be able to recognize pathophysiological derangements associated with pregnant-specific illnesses as well as worsening of premorbid conditions. In addition to the basic components of the preanesthetic assessment, some specific aspects need attention:

- Body mass index—weight gain during pregnancy may contribute to risk of difficult airway, respiratory complications, peripheral neuropathies, and difficult neuraxial access.
- Airway—incidence of difficult airway is 8 to 10 times higher compared to the nonpregnant population.
- Aspiration of gastric contents—it is appropriate to reserve full stomach precautions for patients after 20 weeks' gestation. This is due to a combination of mechanical and hormonal factors. Gastric prophylaxis should be considered prior to the provision of general anesthesia.
- Oxygen reserve—the ability to preoxygenate pregnant patients is compromised due to higher oxygen consumption and reduction of pulmonary functional residual capacity.
- Spinal anatomy—identification of anatomical landmarks at the lumbar spinal level might prove difficult in pregnancy due to an accumulation of fat tissue and edema as well as to a limitation of spinal movement arches. Anatomic abnormalities of the lumbar spine are exaggerated during the third trimester.

- Anemia—physiologic anemia secondary to expanded plasma volume puts the pregnant patient in a risky position in light of an increased risk of peripartum hemorrhage. All patients admitted for delivery must have an updated type and screen.
- Thrombocytopenia—physiologic decreases in platelet counts are usually not a contraindication to regional labor analgesia; however, in particular situations the risk of spinal hematoma may be increased.

3.2.3. Cardiac evaluation for noncardiac procedures

Some patients scheduled for major surgery have a significant risk for adverse cardiovascular events during the perioperative period. Identifying susceptible individuals enables anesthesiologists and surgeons to plan evaluations and interventions to reduce the risk and to better understand and communicate to the patient the risk-benefit ratio of a particular procedure.

A comprehensive preanesthesia evaluation sheds light on the predictors of risk for major cardiac adverse events based on a scoring system such as RCRI and NSQIP. On the other hand, the application of user-friendly algorithms to evaluate patients who need to undergo additional testing and/or interventions prior to the scheduled operation leads to a stepwise approach based on efficiency and patient safety (Box 3.3).

Appropriate use of algorithms to guide the decision-making process depends on knowledge of some basic principles:

- The decision to postpone or delay a procedure depends on whether the benefits of additional testing and/or interventions outweigh the risks of a surgical condition worsened by deferring the operation. In emergencies, risk factors should be controlled perioperatively and the procedure should proceed as planned.
- Additional tests are indicated only if their results would affect surgical or anesthetic management. Proceeding with additional workups or interventions should only occur after a thorough discussion involving anesthesiologist, surgeon, and patient.

Box 3.3 Factors determining stepwise approach of cardiac evaluation for noncardiac surgery

- Emergency surgery
- Presence of acute coronary syndrome
- Risk of major cardiac adverse events
- Functional capacity
- Ability to further test to modify surgical or anesthetic plan

Box 3.4 Information provided by echocardiographic evaluation

- Global left ventricular systolic and diastolic function
- Valve anatomy and function
- Right ventricular anatomy and pulmonary artery pressure
- Pericardial anatomy
- Patients with dyspnea that cannot be explained by pulmonary pathology

- Categorizing surgical risk determines the need for additional evaluations (e.g., a pharmacologic stress test in light of the patient's functional capacity or myocardial revascularization if the tests reveal ischemia).

An electrocardiogram and an echocardiogram should be ordered based on medical history (Box 3.4).

3.2.4. Patients with end-stage liver disease

Patients with end-stage liver disease (ESLD) represent a growing population of individuals who undergo general surgical procedures and transplant interventions. The preanesthesia evaluation in these patients must emphasize identification and optimization of multisystem complications, hemostasis, and fluid status in anticipation of large perioperative fluid shifts and appropriate use of medications with hepatic metabolism and renal excretion.

In addition to general risk stratification, patients with ESLD can be evaluated with the Model for End-stage Liver Disease (MELD) score to predict disease severity (Box 3.5). This score estimates long-term survival and is used to list patients for liver transplantation.

Anesthetic considerations include aspects related to every organ system. It is important to acknowledge that the cardiovascular system is especially affected, as it experiences a state of increased cardiac output and systemic vasodilation. However, the contractile function of the heart can also be compromised due to concurrent coronary artery disease or liver dysfunction. A thorough cardiac evaluation including echocardiographic studies will help to stratify cardiac risk in these individuals.

Box 3.5 MELD score parameters

- Serum creatinine
- Total bilirubin
- PT/INR

An echocardiogram assesses systolic and diastolic function of both ventricles, pericardial sac anatomy, valve function, wall segment abnormalities, and pulmonary artery systolic pressure (PASP). Patients identified as having pulmonary hypertension are candidates for a right heart catheterization. PASP values of 45 to 50 mmHg and/or right ventricular dysfunction adequately screen patients who need catheterization. Mean pulmonary artery pressure higher than 50 mmHg is associated with extremely high perioperative mortality. Finally, based on the preoperative evaluation, patients at significant risk for active coronary artery disease may benefit from an echocardiographic evaluation with a dobutamine challenge.

Further Reading

Blitz JD, Kendale SM, Jain SK, Cuff GE, Kim JT, Rosenberg AD. Preoperative evaluation clinic visit is associated with decreased risk of in-hospital postoperative mortality. *Anesthesiology.* 2016;125(2):280–294.

Cologne KG, Keller DS, Liwanag L, Devaraj B, Senagore AJ. Use of the American College of Surgeons NSQIP Surgical Risk Calculator for laparoscopic colectomy: how good is it and how can we improve it? *J Am Coll Surg.* 2015;220(3):281–286.

Fleisher LA, Fleischmann KE, Auerbach AD, et al. 2014 ACC/AHA guideline on perioperative cardiovascular evaluation and management of patients undergoing noncardiac surgery: a report of the American College of Cardiology/American Heart Association Task Force on practice guidelines. *J Am Coll Cardiol.* 2014;64(22):e77–137.

Friedman LS. Preoperative evaluation of the patient with liver disease. In: Schiff ER, Maddrey WC, Sorrell MF, eds. *Schiff's Diseases of the Liver,* 11th ed. Oxford: Wiley-Blackwell; 2011: ch 13, pp 316–325.

Joint Commission. Medication reconciliation. Sentinel event alert. 2006. https://www.jointcommission.org/assets/1/18/SEA_35.PDF

Sankar A, Johnson SR, Beattie WS, Tait G, Wijeysundera DN. Reliability of the American Society of Anesthesiologists physical status scale in clinical practice. *Br J Anaesth.* 2014;113(3):424–432.

Chapter 4

Anesthesia Care on the Day of Surgery

Claudia F. Clavijo, Mary E. Arthur,
and Efrain Riveros-Perez

4.1. Documentation

4.1.1. Informed consent

Informed consent, the process by which a patient agrees to the anesthetic plan after receiving comprehensive and accurate information, is based on the ethical principle of autonomy. There are three fundamental elements in a valid consent: disclosure, capacity, and voluntariness. Disclosure refers to providing descriptive and accurate information; capacity involves a patient's competence and ability to comprehend. Voluntariness has to do with a patient making a decision that is autonomous and free of coercion. A description of the consent process can be found in 3.1.1.6. Residents should be aware of the policies specific to their institution.

4.1.2. Phases of care assessment and evaluation

Anesthetic care should follow institutional and American Society of Anesthesiologists (ASA) guidelines. The anesthesiologist is responsible for determining the patient's medical status and tailoring an anesthesia plan that is appropriate to the patient's specific needs and condition.

4.1.2.1. Final discussion of plan, completion of physical exam, and documentation update

The following steps are required during the preoperative period:

- Review the medical record and gather information before the patient arrives.
- Interview the patient to obtain medical history, prescribed medications, and personal and family anesthetic history. Patients should also be asked about whether they would accept transfusions of whole blood or blood products should the need arise.

- Perform a physical exam oriented to airway, cardiovascular, respiratory, and neurologic status.
- Order and review relevant laboratory tests, imaging, and consultations (see chapter 3). Previous anesthesia records should be reviewed when available.
- Describe to the patient and family the proposed anesthesia plan and alternatives, if applicable. Be sure to discuss pain management, prophylaxis for postoperative nausea and vomiting, and postoperative care.
- Order preoperative interventions and medications.
- Obtain informed consent before administering any medications that could affect the patient's awareness or memory.
- Ensure these steps are noted in the patient's medical record.

4.1.3. Handwritten requirements

Informed anesthesia consent can be documented on the surgical consent form with a handwritten note or on a separate anesthesia consent form. A standard anesthesia consent form that provides space to write in the precise anesthesia plan may be ideal. Consent forms should be signed and dated by the patient or legal guardian as well as the anesthesia provider before the patient is transported to the surgical suite.

4.1.4. Anesthesia information management systems

The anesthesia information management system (AIMS) is the anesthesia component of the electronic medical record. AIMS collects data in real time during the perioperative period and integrates it into the patient's anesthesia record. AIMS minimizes manual documentation and improves situational awareness (i.e., allowing residents to focus and respond to changes in the patient's status during anesthesia). The system must be highly reliable and its hardware, software, and networks need to be constantly updated and maintained by qualified and dedicated personnel. Although AIMS is not yet available in all institutions, its benefits have been proven, and it is advisable to transition from paper records to AIMS.

4.2. Operating room anesthesia set-up and considerations

4.2.1. Equipment/standard monitors and safety check

Before the patient is brought to the operating room, the resident needs to ensure that equipment including the anesthesia machine is checked and medications are prepared and labeled (Table 4.1 and 4.2).

Table 4.1. Anesthesia room checkout items	
Anesthesia machine	Refer to operator's manual and institutional policies
Monitors	ASA standard monitors and additional monitors as guided by patient condition
Suction	Available and functioning
Surgical table	Functioning and adequate to patient's weight
Airway equipment	Laryngoscope handles and blades, laryngeal mask airway, tracheal tubes, and oral/nasal airways. Difficult airway equipment readily available
Medications	Label with date, time, and concentration. Ensure safe storage (Table 4.2)
Intravenous sets	Regular sets, blood transfusion sets, fluid warmers
Special equipment	Forced air mattresses and equipment. Additional equipment as indicated

Table 4.2. Anesthesia machine check out	
Equipment	Action
Emergency ventilation system	Verify that the auxiliary oxygen cylinder and self-inflating manual ventilation device are available and functioning
Anesthesia delivery system	Turn on and confirm that power is available
Spare oxygen cylinder in the anesthesia machine	Verify that pressure is adequate
Piped gas pressure	Verify that pressure is ≥ 50 PSI
Vaporizers	Verify that vaporizers are filled, filler ports are tightly closed
Gas supply lines	Verify that there are no leaks in the gas supply lines between the flowmeters and the common gas outlet
Oxygen monitor	Verify calibration of the oxygen monitor and check the low oxygen alarm
Scavenging system	Test scavenging system function
Carbon dioxide absorbent	Verify that absorbent is not exhausted
Breathing system	Test breathing system pressure and perform a leak test. Verify that gas flows properly throughout inhalation and exhalation

(Continued)

Table 4.2. Continued	
Equipment	Action
Monitors	Verify availability of the required monitors and set up audible alarms
Suction	Turn on and confirm it is effective to clear the airway
Documentation	Document completion of checkout procedures
Ventilator settings	Confirm ventilator settings and evaluate readiness of equipment to deliver anesthesia care

Modified from the Recommendation for Pre-anesthesia Checkout Procedures, Subcommittee of the American Society of Anesthesiologists Committee on Equipment and Facilities; 2008.

4.2.2. Patient safety considerations

The ASA states that "Qualified anesthesia personnel shall be present in the room throughout the conduct of all general anesthetics, regional anesthesia anesthetics and all monitored anesthesia care." This requirement is based on the very real possibility of rapid changes in patient status during anesthesia and the need for an immediate response to these changes.

During anesthesia, patient oxygenation, ventilation, circulation, and temperature should be evaluated continuously:

- The instruments used should be programmed with low and high thresholds and audible alarms.
- Adequate illumination and exposure of the patient is recommended.
- Continual clinical assessment is also highly encouraged, to include observation of color, chest excursion and reservoir breathing bag, auscultation of breath and heart sounds, and palpation of pulse.
- Be aware of fire and electrical hazards in the operating room. Review ASA updated statements and recommendations in this regard.

4.3. Anesthesia pharmacologic basics

The primary goal of every general anesthetic is to provide amnesia, analgesia, hypnosis, muscle relaxation, and modulation of stress and autonomic nervous activity in response to surgical stimulation. Regional anesthesia produces analgesia, blocks motor function and autonomic responses to regional stimuli, and interferes with central integration of peripheral painful stimulation. General anesthetic medications can be classified in terms of their contribution to the overall goals described earlier and can be used in combination, maximizing their anesthetic effects while minimizing their toxic profiles. When planning for general anesthesia, residents need to know the anesthetic goals in light of the individual patient's characteristics and the needs for both induction and maintenance. It is important to recognize that hypnotic agents have a dose-response profile that allows the anesthesia provider to carefully titrate the dose to cover the spectrum from minimal anesthesia to deep sedation to general anesthesia (Table 4.3).

Currently available inhaled anesthetics include nitrous oxide, isoflurane, sevoflurane, and desflurane. Their pharmacokinetic and pharmacodynamic profiles dictate their anesthetic properties. Choice of inhalational agent depends mainly on patient characteristics, surgical procedure (e.g., neurosurgery), cost, and speed of emergence (desflurane > sevoflurane > isoflurane). Nitrous oxide cannot provide anesthesia as a sole agent due to its extremely high

Table 4.3. Mechanism of action of hypnotic agents used in anesthesia

Medication	Anesthetic goal	Mechanism of action
Benzodiazepines	Sedation, hypnosis, amnesia	GABA receptor antagonism
Propofol	Sedation, hypnosis, amnesia	GABA receptor antagonism
Etomidate	Hypnosis, amnesia	GABA receptor antagonism
Ketamine	Hypnosis, amnesia, analgesia, blunting of autonomic response	NMDA receptor antagonism
Dexmedetomidine	Sedation, analgesia	Alpha-2 adrenergic antagonism
Lidocaine	Analgesia, blunting of autonomic response	Sodium channel block
Opioids	Analgesia, blunting of autonomic response	Opioid receptor antagonism
Muscle relaxants	Muscle relaxation	Nicotine receptor interaction
Inhaled anesthetics	Hypnosis/amnesia/analgesia/autonomic response blunting/muscle relaxation	Interaction with brain cell membranes

minimal alveolar concentration (MAC) and is contraindicated in instances where accumulation of the gas in closed spaces or gas absorption (e.g., pneumothorax, venous air embolism, intestinal obstruction, retinal detachment surgery with gas bubble) is of concern. A detailed discussion of anesthetic pharmacology can be found in specialized anesthesia textbooks.

4.4. Prepping the patient

4.4.1. Pharmacological considerations

Administering anesthetic agents causes a desired effect on the central nervous system at the expense of effects on different organ systems, particularly the cardiovascular and respiratory systems. To be able to predict and control the action of anesthetics on different organ systems, it is critically important to understand the pharmacokinetics and pharmacodynamics of the agents used in anesthesia practice as well as their interactions with the patient's at-home medications. Special preparations and recommendations may be necessary during the preoperative visit to mitigate pharmacological interactions and to optimize the patient's condition to minimize side effects of anesthetic agents.

Unique patient characteristics such as liver and kidney function as well as plasma protein concentration may affect handling of anesthetic drugs. Dose adjustment must be considered in such situations, and, when possible, end-organ effect should be monitored (e.g., bispectral index monitor, end-tidal MAC concentration, hemodynamic variables). Table 4.4 lists recommendations in relation to preoperative administration of medications:

4.4.2. Airway considerations

An essential component of the preanesthesia evaluation is airway assessment. The anesthesiologist can devise a safe and effective plan based on a careful identification of predictors of difficult ventilation and/or intubation. Some patients are seen by an anesthesiologist for the first time on the day of surgery, but even in patients evaluated in the past, a thorough airway exam is mandatory for every case. Components of a comprehensive airway exam (discussed in chapter 1) include review of prior anesthetic records, including a history of a difficult airway, anatomic facial abnormalities, tongue-to-oropharynx ratio (Mallampati score), and objective measurements including mouth opening, thyromental distance, mentohyoid distance, neck circumference, and neck range of motion. Dentition and jaw mobility are also part of the exam.

Table 4.4. Recommendations		
Medication	Recommendation	Risks
Angiotensin converting enzyme inhibitors and receptor blockers	Discontinue the day before surgery	Intraoperative hypotension
Diuretics	Hold on day of surgery	Hypovolemia and electrolyte abnormalities
Warfarin	Stop five days before surgery	Goal to achieve normal INR
Antiplatelet drugs (e.g., clopidogrel, anti-Factor Xa)	Follow American Society of Regional Anesthesia recommendations	Surgical bleeding and spinal hematoma when neuraxial techniques are used
Aspirin	Continue if indicated for cardiac reasons	Surgical bleeding
Low molecular weight heparins	Hold 12 hours preoperatively (prophylactic) or 24 hours (therapeutic)	Bleeding and spinal hematoma
Short-acting insulins	Hold on day of surgery	Hypoglycemia
NPH insulin	Administer half dose on day of surgery	Hypoglycemia
Long-acting insulins	Give usual dose the day of surgery	Monitor blood sugar perioperatively
Oral diabetic medications	Hold on day of surgery	Monitor glycemic level

If the airway exam is concerning, the ASA difficult airway algorithm can be used to guide the decision-making process. The anesthesia team has to make a decision on an awake versus post-induction intubation, suppression of spontaneous ventilation, and use of special devices. The resident must be familiar with the various devices including direct laryngoscopes with different blades, laryngeal mask airways, oral and nasal airways, videolaryngoscopes, fiber optic bronchoscopes, elastic bougies, and tube exchangers. Recognizing when a surgical airway is indicated and when to call for help is an important attribute for all anesthesiology residents.

Table 4.5. American Society of Anesthesiologists standard monitors		
Physiologic function	Physical signs	Monitor
Oxygenation	Skin and mucosal color	Pulse oxymeter and oxygen analyzer
Ventilation	Breath sound, chest movement	End-tidal CO_2, minute ventilation
Circulation	Heart sounds, pulse	Electrocardiograph, noninvasive blood pressure
Temperature	Skin temperature	Temperature probe

4.4.3. Monitoring considerations

The decision to employ specific monitoring techniques depends on ASA standards, surgery-related factors, patient comorbidities, and clinical condition (Table 4.5).

Guidelines:

- Use invasive blood pressure monitoring in cases where hemodynamic swings are poorly tolerated; when hypotensive or hypertensive episodes are life-threatening (e.g., active coronary artery disease, critical aortic stenosis, brain aneurysm) or when frequent blood sampling is anticipated (metabolic, hemoglobin levels, electrolytes, and arterial blood gases).
- Use central venous access in cases of difficult peripheral venous access, for the administration of vasoactive medications, in cases where there is a high-risk of venous air embolism (multi-orifice catheters), and as a conduit to advance a venous pacemaker electrode or a pulmonary artery catheter.
- Place a Foley catheter in long procedures or when expecting large fluid shifts.
- Use a neuromuscular function monitor whenever a muscle relaxant is used.
- Consider sophisticated monitoring techniques such as transesophageal echocardiography, monitors of anesthetic depth, and neuromonitoring in specific cases.

4.4.4. Ventilation considerations

General anesthesia reduces functional residual capacity and results in atelectasis in up to 90% of patients. Most patients under general anesthesia require intraoperative mechanical ventilation. Optimizing intraoperative mechanical ventilation can reduce the incidence of postoperative pulmonary complications and improve patient outcomes. The ventilators on anesthesia machines

Table 4.6. Modes of mechanical ventilation in anesthesia machines

Name	Description	Variables
CMV (controlled mechanical ventilation)	Ventilator delivers 100% of breaths. Pressure control with volume guarantee is a variation pressure adjusted to set tidal volume	Control: Pressure or volume
		Trigger: Time
		Cycle: Time
		Limit: Pressure
PSV (pressure support ventilation)	Ventilator triggered by patient, pressurizes airway to deliver tidal volume. Depends on patient's respiratory drive and can be used for weaning	Control: Pressure
		Trigger: Pressure or flow
		Cycle: When flow reaches 25% of peak
		Limit: None
SIMV (synchronized intermittent mandatory ventilation)	Ventilator delivers a breath at a set frequency and allows patient to breathe without support. It is used in combination with PSV	Control: Pressure or volume
		Trigger: Time
		Cycle: Time
		Limit: Pressure

increasingly allow modes of ventilation with most, but not all, of the capabilities of ventilators used in the intensive care unit. Basic ventilator modes are distinguished by four important variables: control (driving variable), trigger (inspiratory initiation), cycle (switch from inspiration to expiration), and limit (forced cycling) (Table 4.6).

Pressure steadily increases during inspiration, as gas (typically at a constant flow rate) fills the lungs. During expiration, pressure drops quickly as the chest and diaphragm passively recoil (Figure 4.1).

The ventilator quickly reaches the set pressure and maintains it throughout the breath. This requires an increased respiratory flow at the onset of the breath and a small delay for the ventilator to reach the target pressure. Expiratory flows are passive and follow the same waveform as in volume control (Figure 4.2).

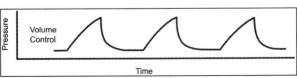

Figure 4.1. Volume-controlled ventilation (VCV)

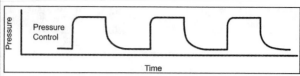

Figure 4.2. Pressure-controlled ventilation (PCV)

The patient initiates each pressure-controlled breath by generating negative pressure (note the downward deflections prior to the pressure support), and thus inspiratory timing is dependent on patient effort (Figure 4.3).

A volume-controlled breath is delivered with each inspiratory effort. If the patient fails to initiate a breath after a set interval, however, the ventilator will deliver a volume-controlled breath regardless (Figure 4.4).

The choice of ventilator should be based on patient factors, surgical procedure, and available technology. For many healthy patients who undergo routine surgery, any mode of ventilation may be used to provide effective and safe intraoperative ventilation. The anesthesia provider sets parameters specific to each patient, procedure, or mode of ventilation (Table 4.7).

During mechanical ventilation, respiratory mechanics should be monitored. Peak airway pressure reflects airway resistance, whereas plateau pressure depends on elastic properties of the lung, chest wall, and diaphragm. The goal is to keep peak pressure below 40 cm H_2O and plateau pressure below 30 cm H_2O. Pressure:time, flow:volume and pressure:volume graphs are useful to monitor mechanics of the respiratory system.

Recruitment maneuvers consisting of the application of a brief (6- to 8-second) high level of continuous positive airway pressure will reverse atelectasis and improve oxygenation. During a recruitment maneuver, an inspiratory pressure of 30 to 40 cm H_2O is required to expand the anesthesia-induced atelectatic lung. Protective mechanical ventilation using low target tidal volume calculated based on the ideal body weight rather than actual body weight and low levels of positive end-expiratory pressure should

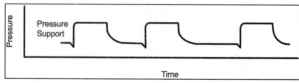

Figure 4.3. Pressure-support ventilation (PSV)

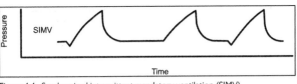

Figure 4.4. Synchronized intermittent mandatory ventilation (SIMV)

be used in patients requiring mechanical ventilation under general anesthesia.

4.4.5. Positioning considerations

Positioning for a surgical procedure is a shared responsibility of the operating room team—the anesthesia provider, surgeon, and operating room nurses. Optimal positioning of the surgical patient balances the need for adequate surgical exposure with the goal of preventing injury (Table 4.8, Figures 5–10).

To achieve optimal positioning, ensure:

- Adequate arterial supply and venous outflow are maintained to all body parts.
- Nerves are protected from undue pressure or stretching.
- Bony prominences are padded.
- Circulatory and respiratory systems are minimally compromised.
- Maximum surgical field exposure is achieved.

Table 4.7. Ventilator settings	
Tidal volume (TV)	6–8 mL/kg is recommended
Respiratory rate (RR)	Typically 8–16 breaths/min to keep $ETCO_2$ around 40 mmHg
Inspiratory to expiratory ratio	Usually 1:2 or 1:2.5. Increase if airway obstruction occurs
Positive end-expiratory pressure	Most patients benefit from 5 cm H_2O
Pressure limit	Maximum pressure that causes cycling
Peak inspiratory pressure	Affected by airway resistance
Pressure support	Adjusted according to RR and TV
Minimum RR	Backup mode to trigger-controlled breath
Pressure or flow trigger	Negative inspiratory pressure or increase in flow to trigger
Inspired oxygen fraction (FiO_2)	Start with 1.0, titrate down according to O_2 saturation

Table 4.8. Prevention of positioning risks

Position	Risks	Maneuvers
Supine See Figure 4.5.	Brachial plexus injury	Abduct arms <90° Hand/forearm neutral
Trendelenburg See Figure 4.6	Patient sliding cephalad	Nonsliding mattress
	Upper airway edema and increase in central venous return	Judicious fluid management
	Decreased vital capacity and functional residual capacity	Adjust ventilator settings
Prone See Figure 4.7	Spine injury during rotation	Maintain alignment during rotation
	Pressure on eyes, breasts and male genitals	Check pressure points
	Increased abdominal pressure	Leave abdomen free of pressure
	Cervical spine stress	Keep >2 fingerbreadths between chin and chest
Lithotomy See Figure 4.8	Torsion of lumbar spine	Move legs simultaneously
	Nerve injury due to stretching	Keep hips flexed 80°–100°, legs abducted 30°–45°
	Nerve compression	Ensure adequate padding of extremities
	Finger crush injury	Keep extremities away from table hinge points
Lateral See Figure 4.9	Cervical spine and brachial plexus injury	Keep head in neutral position and place shoulder roll
	Peripheral nerve compression	Pad arms, knees, and ankles
Sitting/ beach chair See Figure 4.10	Brachial plexus injury	Support arms with adequate padding
	Venous air embolism	Adequate monitoring
	Cervical spine injury	Keep head in neutral position
	↓ Mean arterial pressure (MAP)	Aggressively treat blood pressure Correct MAP for hydrostatic gradient
	↓ Cerebral perfusion pressure	Keep MAP >70 mmHg ↑ ETCO$_2$ from 30 to 45 mmHg
	Cerebral desaturation	↑ FiO$_2$

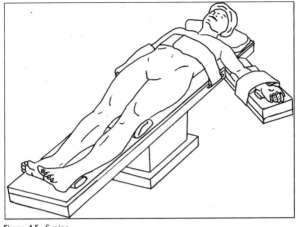

Figure 4.5. Supine

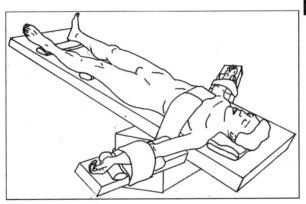

Figure 4.6. Tredelenburg

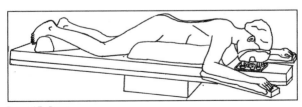

Figure 4.7. Prone

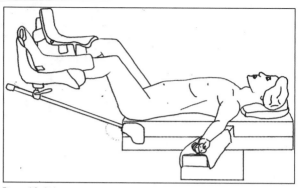

Figure 4.8. Lithotomy

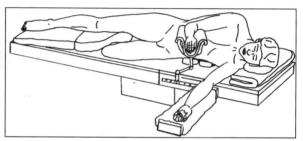

Figure 4.9. Lateral

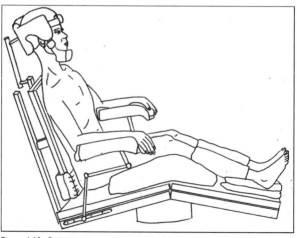

Figure 4.10. Sitting

For all positions:
- Apply padding to heels, elbows, knees, and occiput.
- Pad IV tubing and stopcocks touching the skin.

In the sitting position for every 1 cm difference between the cuff and the auditory meatus, MAP would be 0.77 mmHg lower (i.e., 1 mmHg for every 1.25 cm). When using an arterial line, measure blood pressure at the level of the brain (i.e., zero the transducer at the external auditory meatus). Increase $ETCO_2$ 30 to 45 mmHg to prevent cerebral vasoconstriction.

4.4.6. Positioning complications

4.4.6.1. Peripheral neuropathy
- Sensory/motor neuropathy
- Typically transient
- Patient follow-up is important
- Consider neurology consultation
- A baseline EMG will help determine a preexisting nerve injury (changes in EMG activity do not appear until two to three weeks after a nerve injury)
- Consider physical therapy for best outcomes

4.4.6.2. Upper extremity injuries
4.4.6.2.1. Ulnar nerve injury
Ulnar nerve injury is the most common problem in anesthetized patients.
- Compression between the medial epicondyle and the arm board or bed
- Loss of sensation of the lateral portion of hand and inability to abduct or oppose the fifth finger

4.4.6.2.2. Brachial plexus injury
- Occurs when brachial plexus is stretched or compressed between the clavicle and first rib
- Manifestations depend on which nerves are injured
  - Median nerve: inability to oppose thumb
  - Axillary nerve: inability to abduct the arm
  - Musculoskeletal nerve: inability to flex the forearm
  - Radial nerve: wrist drop
  - Ulnar nerve: loss of sensation of the lateral portion of hand and inability to abduct or oppose the fifth finger

4.4.6.3. Lower extremity injuries

4.4.6.3.1. Common peroneal nerve injury

Common peroneal nerve injury is most common in the lithotomy position.

- Results in foot drop and a loss of dorsal extension of toes

4.4.6.3.2. Sciatic nerve

- Results from excessive flexion of the hips
- Weakness in all muscles below the knee and foot drop.

4.4.6.3.3. Femoral nerve

- Trapping under the inguinal ligament from extreme flexion and abduction of thighs
- Decreased knee jerk, loss of hip flexion, and knee extension

4.4.6.3.4. Saphenous nerve

- Injured when the medial tibial condyle is compressed by leg support in lithotomy position
- Paresthesia along medial and anteromedial aspect of the calf

4.4.6.3.5. Anterior tibial nerve

- Injured when feet are plantar flexed for extended periods of time in the sitting and prone position
- Manifests as foot drop

4.4.6.3.6. Obturator nerve

- Damaged during excessive flexion of the thigh to the groin
- Results in inability to adduct the leg and diminished sensation along medial aspect of the thigh

4.4.7. Eye injury

- Corneal abrasion is the most common eye injury
- Postoperative blindness
- Risks include intraoperative hypotension, prone position, and anemia
- Etiology includes optic neuropathy and or retinal vessel occlusion
- Requires immediate consultation with an ophthalmologist

The ASA Practice Advisory for the Prevention of Perioperative Peripheral Neuropathies encourages anesthesia providers to ascertain whether patients can comfortably tolerate the anticipated operative position during the preoperative assessment. A simple postoperative assessment of extremity nerve function may facilitate early recognition of peripheral neuropathies. Documentation of specific perioperative positioning actions may be useful for continuous improvement processes and may result in (a) focusing the practitioner's attention on relevant aspects of patient positioning and (b) providing information on positioning strategies that leads to improvements in patient care.

Further Reading

American Society of Anesthesiologists. Standard for Basic Anesthetic Monitoring. Approved by House of Delegates on October 21, 1986; last amended on October 20, 2010; and last affirmed on October 28, 2015.

American Society of Anesthesiologists Task Force on Prevention of Perioperative Peripheral Neuropathies. Practice advisory for the prevention of perioperative peripheral neuropathies: an updated report by the American Society of Anesthesiologists Task Force on prevention of perioperative peripheral neuropathies. *Anesthesiology.* 2011;114(4):741.

Apfelbaum JL, Hagberg CA, Caplan RA, et al. Practice guidelines for management of the difficult airway: an updated report by the American Society of Anesthesiologists Task Force on Management of the Difficult Airway. *Anesthesiology.* 2013;118(2):251–270.

Ball L, Dameri M, Pelosi P. Modes of mechanical ventilation for the operating room. *Best Pract Res Clin Anaesthesiol.* 2015; 29(3):285–299.

Barash PG, Cullen BF, Stoelting RK. *Clinical Anesthesia,* 7th ed. Philadelphia: Wolters Kluwer/Lippincott Williams & Wilkins; 2014.

Chilkoti G, Wadhwa R, Saxena AK. Technological advances in perioperative monitoring: current concepts and clinical perspectives. *J Anaesthesiol Clin Pharmacol.* 2015;31(1): 14–24.

Chu LF, Fuller A. *Manual of Clinical Anesthesiology.* Philadelphia: Lippincott Williams & Wilkins; 2012.

Hedenstierna G, Edmark L. The effects of anesthesia and muscle paralysis on the respiratory system. *Intensive Care Med.* 2005;31(10):1327–1335.

Simula DV, Mueller JT, Anesthesia information management systems. In: Murray MJ, Rose SH, Wedel DJ, Wass CT, Harrison BA, Mueller JT, & Trentman TL, eds. *Faust's Anesthesiology Review E-Book: Expert Consult.* Elsevier Health Sciences; 2014: ch 251, pp 593–594.

Van den Berg JP, Vereecke HE, Proost JH, et al. Pharmacokinetic and pharmacodynamic interactions in anaesthesia: a review of current knowledge and how it can be used to optimize anaesthetic drug administration. *Br J Anaesth.* 2017;118(1):44–57.

Wanderer JP, Rathmell JP. Perioperative medication management. *Anesthesiology.* 2017;126(1):A21.

Welch MB. Patient positioning for surgery and anesthesia in adults In: Wahr JA, Crowley M, eds. 2017. UptoDate. Available from https://www.uptodate.com/contents/patient-positioning-for-surgery-and-anesthesia-in-adults

Chapter 5

Fundamentals of Anesthetic Care

Claudia F. Clavijo and Efrain Riveros-Perez

5.1. Anesthesia care basics

5.1.1. Surgical time-out

The World Health Organization and Joint Commission require that hospitals implement a time-out before surgery starts. A time out allows team members—surgery, anesthesia, and nursing—to discuss relevant safety concerns and particular aspects of the procedure. This initiative promotes communication among team members; improves anesthesia safety practices; and reduces surgical infections, errors, and deaths. This practice is done in a single step or is divided into three parts: sign in (Box 5.1), time out (Box 5.2), and sign out (Box 5.3).

Sign in, or "huddle"—done before induction of anesthesia—reviews important aspects of the procedure.

5.1.2. Induction

Induction of anesthesia is the loss of consciousness after the administration of anesthetic agents, either intravenous (IV) or inhalational. The most common IV induction agents are propofol, etomidate, and ketamine. A combination of benzodiazepines and opioids can be used in some situations. Sevoflorane is commonly used as an inhalational induction agent in children, in patients with poor venous access, or when maintaining spontaneous ventilation during induction is preferable. During induction, patients lose the ability to maintain a patent airway and independent ventilatory function. Loss of eyelash reflex is commonly used as an endpoint of appropriate induction dose.

Throughout this transition from awake to anesthetized state, a patent airway must be maintained. Positive pressure ventilation may be required due to depressed spontaneous ventilation. Before induction, the anesthesiologist should decide how the airway will be secured—by endotracheal tube or supraglottic airway device—based on patient and surgical factors such as length of

Box 5.1 Sign in or "huddle"

- Patient identification—patient should be asked to participate whenever possible
- Procedure to be performed
- Consents—signed for the intended procedure
- Site of the procedure—site should be marked. A written alternative or institutional protocol to ensure the correct site identification should be used when marking is not technically or anatomically possible.
- Known allergies—should be listed
- Anticipated difficult airway or high risk of aspiration
- Anticipated blood loss—discuss risk of major blood loss (>500 mL or 7 mL/kg in children)
- Blood products—patient acceptance or refusal for whole blood, blood products
- Code status

the procedure, patient positioning, and surgical site. If intubation is required, a neuromuscular blocking agent may be used. Rapid sequence induction is recommended if the risk of aspiration during induction is high. Cardiovascular function needs constant vigilance since it could also be affected by induction medications. Induction agent selection and dosing should be tailored to patient's age, weight, and clinical condition (Table 5.1).

Box 5.2 Time out: Performed before skin incision

Confirm:
- Name and role of all team members
- Patient, procedure to be performed and laterality, if applicable
- Anticipated surgical time, difficult or critical portions of the procedure, and anticipated blood loss
- Whether antibiotic prophylaxis has been received within 60 minutes prior to incision
- Anesthesia concerns
- Nursing confirms sterility of equipment and availability of all required instruments
- Availability of imaging if applicable
- Anticipated destination of patient after the procedure
- If more than one procedure will be performed by a different surgeon, a second time out should be done

> Box 5.3 Sign out: Performed before patient leaves
> the operating room
>
> Critical aspects to be reviewed:
> - Procedure has been recorded
> - Correct needle, sponge and instrument count
> - How specimens were labeled and what will be their final desti-
>   nation. Problems or difficulties during the procedure that need
>   to be addressed
> - Important information to be transmitted to the next care team

5.1.3. Maintenance

After induction, inhalational agents or a continuous infusion of IV
medications are used to keep the patient unconscious. Minimal alveolar concentration (MAC) is the alveolar concentration of a volatile agent that prevents movement in 50% of healthy volunteers
after a given surgical stimulation (i.e., skin incision). The concentration of the inhalational agent is measured with a gas analyzer and is
displayed on the monitor. The expired end-tidal concentration of
the inhalational agent can be used as a surrogate measure for the
amount of agent reaching the central nervous system. MAC varies
among inhalational agents and is affected by patient and surgical
factors. An IV infusion of propofol can also be utilized for maintenance with or without an opioid infusion. Infusion pumps are used
to safely administer the IV agent. Patient characteristics such as
age, gender and weight are factored in the infusion dose. If total intravenous anesthesia is used for maintenance, the anesthesiologist
should consider monitoring anesthesia depth with processed elec-
troencephalography (EEG). The use of neuromuscular blockade
throughout the procedure should be discussed with the surgical
team. Although some procedures require constant neuromuscular
blockade, in others, these agents are contraindicated or should
be avoided. An example is when a patient needs motor evoked
potentials or electromyography monitoring.

Table 5.1. Common induction agents		
Induction agent	Induction dose	Special considerations
Propofol	1.5–2.5 mg/kg	Expected vascular dilatation and hypotension
Etomidate	0.2–0.3 mg/kg	Concern for adrenal suppression. Myoclonus
Ketamine	1–2 mg/kg	Sympathomimetic discharge and myocardial depression

Besides keeping the patient unconscious and immobile during maintenance, the anesthesiologist should constantly evaluate airway patency; optimize respiratory parameters to maintain oxygen saturation and lung protection; maintain appropriate cardiac output, fluid balance, and tissue perfusion; and provide analgesia specific to the individual's needs. Antiemetic medications are also provided before emergence. Requirements of analgesia should be constantly evaluated throughout the surgical procedure since different levels of stimulation may require adjustment of the analgesics provided.

5.1.4. Emergence and extubation

Once surgery is over, anesthetics are no longer required. A plan for extubation that accounts for patient status and surgical needs should be in place. Inhalational or IV infusions should be turned off. The endotracheal tube can be removed after suction of oropharyngeal secretions and when extubation criteria have been met. In certain situations, deep extubation may be preferable to avoid coughing and extreme elevations in blood pressure. Emergency medications should always be available to treat an unexpected airway or hemodynamic events that may occur during or after extubation, such as laryngospasm or hemodynamic instability. As patients are waking up, they may become agitated. Enough personnel should be available to keep patients from falling or removing lines or drains.

5.2. Patient management

5.2.1. Regional block for acute pain management

One of the anesthetic goals is to ensure intra and postoperative analgesia. Pain control helps modulate stress and inflammatory responses. Analgesia should be provided in a multimodal approach to maximize the desired effect while mitigating the side effects of each individual strategy. Regional techniques including neuraxial and peripheral blocks have gained popularity among anesthesia providers over the past decade. The introduction of ultrasound technology has contributed to the widespread use of peripheral nerve blocks. Knowledge of nerve anatomy and training in the use of emerging technologies is necessary to guarantee safe use regional techniques.

Spinal analgesia with intrathecal morphine provides pain control for at least 24 hours in lower extremity surgery and in selected lower abdominal procedures. The main side effects associated with this technique are respiratory depression and pruritus. Continuous monitoring of respiratory function is recommended and cautious use of supplemental opioids, oral or parenteral, for the first 12 hours is advised. Preoperative placement of an epidural catheter is another alternative to spinal morphine. Epidural catheters have the advantage of allowing administration of a low concentration of local anesthetic and/or opioid infusions for as long as 72 hours; however, some surgeons are concerned with potential delayed ambulation. When an epidural catheter is left in place, it is recommended that the infusion of choice is started only when the patient is hemodynamically stable close to the end of the procedure, when the blood loss has been finally estimated.

Peripheral nerve blocks can be performed by anatomical landmarks or nerve stimulation and with ultrasound guidance. The latter technique is preferred and is part of residency training. The anesthesiology resident should be familiar with nerve anatomy and the basics of ultrasound. Indications and contraindications of nerve blocks must be acknowledged before performing the procedure. Table 5.2 shows the most common peripheral nerve blocks, their indications, and special considerations.

Table 5.2. Indications for nerve blocks		
Nerve block	Indications	Special considerations
Interscalene brachial plexus	Surgery of shoulder and arm	Phrenic nerve block. Spares ulnar nerve
Supraclavicular brachial plexus	Surgery of upper extremity distal to shoulder	Risk of pneumothorax
Infraclavicular brachial plexus	Surgery of upper extremity distal to the axilla	Separate injections over brachial plexus chords
Axillary brachial plexus	Surgery distal to elbow	Risk of hematoma
Distal blocks of median, ulnar and radial nerves	Hand surgery	Separate blocks
Lumbar plexus block	Surgery of thigh, patella and knee arthroscopy. Analgesia for knee/hip arthroplasty	Risk of spinal/ epidural injection and hematoma formation
Femoral nerve block	Surgery of thigh, patella and knee arthroscopy. Analgesia for knee/hip arthroplasty	Safe and easy to perform. May need postoperative sciatic block
Sciatic block	Lower extremity surgery below the knee	Might need combination with femoral nerve block
Popliteal nerve block	Surgery of foot and ankle	May need supplemental saphenous or femoral nerve block

5.2.2. Intraoperative awareness

General anesthesia is provided to millions of patients worldwide each year. Despite the safety profile of general anesthetics, the mechanism of action of multiple agents is still a matter of debate, limiting complete control over side effects and adequate titration to effect in some cases. One of the most dreaded complications of general anesthesia—intraoperative recall and awareness—has gained wide media attention. Although the incidence of awareness is as low as 1 per 1,000 anesthetics, the consequences can be devastating for the affected individual.

Preventing awareness starts with identification of risk factors (Box 5.4). Monitoring strategies may help reduce the risk and liability implications. Intraoperative monitoring modalities should combine complementary techniques, including clinical observation (e.g., patient movement), multisystem monitors (e.g., hemodynamic variables, capnogram), and brain function monitoring (processed EEG) such as the bispectral index (BIS). Use of this monitor is not recommended for all general anesthetics but should be considered in high-risk cases. Finally, monitoring of end-tidal concentration of halogenated agents is comparable to the BIS monitor to reduce the risk of intraoperative awareness when inhaled anesthesia is utilized.

When a case of intraoperative awareness is identified, a stepwise approach based on acknowledgement of the patient's distress and psychological support is warranted. Quality improvement

---

Box 5.4 Risk factors for intraoperative awareness

Factors related to procedure:
- Cardiac surgery
- Obstetric surgery
- Emergency operations
- Trauma procedures

Factors related to the patient:
- Chronic use of opioids and benzodiazepines
- Alcohol consumption
- Severe anxiety
- History of awareness
- Difficult airway

Factors related to equipment:
- Malfunction
- Misuse

programs at the institutional level must be put in place to prevent future cases (Box 5.5).

5.2.3. Difficult airway algorithms

A central component of anesthesia practice is airway management. Anticipation of difficulty with ventilation and/or intubation should trigger a sequence of actions leading to safe access to the airway to maintain oxygenation and ventilation in temporary and definitive ways. A stepwise approach to airway management is highly recommended. Different algorithms that include multiple airway devices help the practitioner to walk through an easy-to-remember decision-making process. Just like navigating through algorithms, performing dry runs is equally important to prepare for the actual event when it happens and to achieve the mental speed needed in emergencies. We recommend the difficult airway algorithm of the American Society of Anesthesiologists as a tool to help the clinician tackle challenging airway cases.

5.2.4. Fluid management

Fluid administration during the perioperative period is necessary to maintain intravascular volume and ventricular preload. Continuous

---

Box 5.5 Intraoperative awareness

Preventive measures:

- Check patency of IV catheters and end-tidal concentration of inhaled agent
- Consider premedication with benzodiazepines
- Avoid muscle paralysis when not required by surgical procedure
- When using halogenated agents, keep MAC above 0.7
- Use benzodiazepines when light anesthesia is necessary

Management strategies:

- Address the issue immediately when a patient relates awareness
- Listen carefully and respectfully to patient's account
- Sympathize with the patient
- Reassure the patient and apologize
- Tell the patient that you will start a quality improvement program for the incident
- Notify the surgical team
- Document interview in the chart
- Consult psychology for evaluation and support

fluid losses in the form of urine output and other difficult to measure sources (insensible losses) make it reasonable to administer fluids to maintain a neutral balance. The traditional approach calculates the amount of fluids to be administered based on fasting hours, maintenance needs, and anticipated losses depending on the type of surgery. With this approach, overestimation of maintenance fluids can lead to fluid overload in patients with borderline cardiac function. However, in long procedures with large mucosal exposure, the anesthesiologist might underestimate fluid loss and the patient could be at risk for hypovolemia.

A more reasonable approach is goal-directed therapy. With this technique, stroke volume optimization is set as a goal based on the Frank-Starling principle that links end-diastolic and end-systolic volumes. However, in most instances, stroke volume is not routinely measured, and a surrogate of fluid responsiveness such as pulse pressure variation may become necessary. Trans-thoracic echocardiographic assessment of response to fluid challenges is another alternative when this technology is available.

Recent data have shown that a restrictive fluid approach is associated with a significant reduction in minor and major postoperative complications in selected surgical populations. On the other hand, a more liberal approach may reduce the incidence of postoperative nausea and vomiting (PONV) and improve tissue oxygenation. It seems reasonable to recommend liberal administration of fluids in procedures without significant tissue trauma and endothelial dysfunction, whereas in major surgery, outcomes might be better with a restrictive approach. Regarding the type of fluid employed during surgery, no significant difference between crystalloids and colloids has been found in most surgical settings. Moreover, in trauma patients, colloid administration may actually increase mortality in trauma patients.

5.2.5. Transfusion therapy

Hemostatic function is a physiological mechanism necessary to limit bleeding during surgery. Cellular and humoral factors involved in hemostasis are part of the complex network of inflammation, immunomodulation, and tissue repair. Oxygen transport to peripheral tissues in the context of increased metabolic demand associated with surgical stress is critical to maintain aerobic metabolism. The hematocrit level determines viscosity and rheologic properties of blood that affect oxygen delivery at the capillary level. Transfusion of blood products to restore hemoglobin concentration and hemostatic function is associated with side effects and complications that range from mild fever to life-threatening conditions such as severe hemolytic reactions (Box 5.6).

Box 5.6 Complications of blood transfusion

Infectious:
- Bacterial contamination
- Transmission of disease (HIV, hepatitis, CMV)

Noninfectious nonhemolytic:
- Metabolic complications (hyperkalemia, citrate toxicity)
- Disseminated intravascular coagulation
- Circulatory overload
- Febrile reactions
- Allergic reactions
- Transfusion-related acute lung injury
- Hemolytic transfusion reactions

The decision to transfuse blood components must be based on sound clinical judgment. Utilization of hemoglobin level thresholds to trigger transfusion of packed red blood cells (pRBC) may lead to unnecessary transfusion therapy in some cases. The presence of significant ongoing surgical bleeding, evidence of end-organ damage due to blood loss, low hemoglobin levels (e.g., 7g/dL) in patients with cardiopulmonary and cerebrovascular disease, and metabolic acidosis due to anemic hypoxia are possible indications for administration of pRBC.

When significant blood loss is anticipated or there is an intraoperative indication for transfusion, type and screen and/or cross-match must be ordered.

- Typing consists of mixing type O red cells with the patient's serum to identify the blood group.
- Screening for common antibodies is then done by mixing commercially available red cells exhibiting the antibodies with the patient's serum.
- Cross-matching consists of exposing the red cells to be transfused to the patient's serum. The latter test is the final mandatory step before initiating the blood transfusion.

In exceptional emergencies such as in trauma cases, where there is no time to complete the process of type and cross-match, the first units administered are O negative after which the massive transfusion protocol is activated. An early switch to cross-matched blood is always recommended. When massive bleeding occurs, early concomitant administration of fresh frozen plasma and platelets is indicated. Cryoprecipitate is administered when hypofibrinogenemia is documented.

5.2.6. Hypoxemia

Support of respiratory function during anesthesia includes maintaining oxygenation, ventilation, and elastic/dynamic mechanical respiratory variables within physiological levels. Hypoxemia is defined as arterial oxygen saturation lower than 90% at sea level. The ability of the lungs to oxygenate is a more useful concept, as it refers to the physiological mechanisms that maintain normal arterial pressure of oxygen at the lowest inspired oxygen fraction, ideally at room air. Hypoxemia and poor ability of the lung to oxygenate may result from five different mechanisms (Box 5.7) that can occur alone or in combination. Treatment includes administration of supplemental oxygen and implementation of therapeutic maneuvers to address one or more of the five pathological mechanisms.

When a patient exhibits changes in oxygenation or full-blown hypoxemia, the anesthesiologist must follow a systematic approach. Initially, a quick assessment of the monitors for quality of plethysmography, presence of arrhythmias, hemodynamic status, and changes in capnography should be done, followed by switching to manual ventilation to "feel" the compliance of the circuit/tube/respiratory system and bilateral chest auscultation. At this point, a list of differential diagnoses based on physical and monitor signs must be ruled out, thinking in terms of the five causes of hypoxemia. The resultant possible culprits at the end of this diagnostic exercise should be treated accordingly.

5.2.7. Electrolyte abnormalities

Homeostasis of fluid and electrolyte concentrations in body compartments is necessary for adequate organ function. Fluid status, electrolyte concentration, and acid-base equilibrium interact in a coordinated fashion to preserve cellular metabolic functions and transmembrane electric potential and function of excitable

---

Box 5.7 Pathophysiological mechanisms of hypoxemia

Low alveolar oxygen pressure
- Low barometric pressure (high altitude)
- Low inspired oxygen fraction
- Hypoventilation

Alteration of diffusion (pulmonary edema, pulmonary fibrosis)

Pulmonary and extra pulmonary shunt fraction

Ventilation-to-perfusion mismatch

Low oxygen delivery in the presence of shunt

tissues as well as mechanical function of the cardiovascular system. Virtually any electrolyte abnormality leads to deranged function at different organ levels; however, sodium, potassium, and calcium imbalances deserve special attention in anesthesiology and critical care. Determination of time course, etiology, and clinical manifestations of electrolyte changes is needed to plan an effective therapy (Table 5.3).

5.2.8. PONV prevention

PONV occurs in up to 25% of patients after surgery. PONV negatively affects patient satisfaction and hospital costs. Quality improvement programs in surgical units address this important outcome and aim to prevent it. Prevention of PONV starts with identification of high-risk patients, use of multimodal antiemetic therapies, and avoidance of factors known to trigger this

Table 5.3. Clinically relevant electrolyte disorders		
Electrolyte abnormality	Causes	Treatment
Hypernatremia	Loss of water (diabetes insipidus, diarrhea, vomiting)	Restore fluid volume. Slow replacement of hypotonic solutions (if necessary). DDAVP for DI
Hyponatremia	Excess water concentration: Syndrome of inadequate secretion of antiduiretic hormone (SIADH). Excess sodium loss: Cerebral salt wasting syndrome (CSW)	SIADH: Fluid restriction. CSW: Normal or hypertonic sodium chloride, fludrocortisone.
Hyperkalemia	Increased intake, impaired excretion, potassium shift from intracellular compartment	Calcium chloride if EKG changes. Insulin:Dextrose solution, furosemide, salbutamol, bicarbonate, hemodialysis. Kaeyexalate in chronic cases
Hypokalemia	Transcellular shift, poor intake, metabolic and respiratory alkalosis	Potassium replacement. Caution with speed of infusion. Low concentration solution if administered peripherally
Hypocalcemia	Calcium depletion, alkalosis, renal insufficiency, citrate toxicity	Calcium chloride or gluconate. Monitor ionized calcium
Hypercalcemia	Hyperparathyroidism, chemotherapy, bone tumors	Calcium replacement

Box 5.8 Risk factors for postoperative nausea and vomiting

Factors related to medication use:

• Opioid use

• Neostigmine

• Nitrous oxide and halogenated agents

Factors related to the patient:

• Female gender

• History of postoperative nausea and vomiting

• History of motion sickness

• Nonsmoker

Factors related to the procedure:

• Duration of surgery

• Type of surgery (ear, gynecological, strabismus, breast, shoulder)

complication. Pain control and adequate hydration are also effective preventive measures (Box 5.8).

Pharmacologic interventions are effective when agents binding different receptors are used in combination. It is important for the anesthesiologist to know in detail the pharmacokinetic and pharmacodynamic profiles as well as the side effects associated with their use (Table 5.4).

5.2.9. Extubation criteria and delayed emergence

A comprehensive anesthetic plan should anticipate emergence, recovery, and postoperative destination. The decision to extubate the patient in the operating room depends on factors ranging from respiratory function to metabolic status and hemodynamic stability (Box 5.9). If the anesthesiologist deems it appropriate to keep the patient intubated and transfer him or her to the intensive care unit, arrangements should be made to safely transport the patient.

Table 5.4. Treatment of postoperative nausea and vomiting	
5-HT3 receptor antagonists	Ondansetron, granisetron, tropisetron
Antihistamine	Promethazine
Anti-cholinergic	Scopolamine
Steroids	Dexamethasone
Dopaminergic antagonists	Droperidol, metoclopramide, domperidone

Box 5.9 Extubation criteria

Neurological parameters:
- Patient responsiveness, follows commands
- Ability to protect the airway

Respiratory parameters:
- Adequate oxygenation (SaO_2 >92% with FiO_2 <0.3)
- Normal or baseline CO_2 and acid base status
- Respiratory rate <25 breaths/min
- Tidal volume >5 mL/kg
- Vital capacity >10 mL/kg
- Nonlaborious respiratory pattern

Other parameters:
- Normothermia
- Hemodynamic stability
- Adequate metabolic profile (electrolytes, blood sugar)

These provisions include ensuring hemodynamic and respiratory stability and using a transport monitor and a source of oxygen as well as setting up airway equipment and emergency medications. A complete hand-off report should be delivered to the physician in the critical care unit.

In some instances, emergence from general anesthesia takes longer than would be expected based on the pharmacologic profile of the agents employed (Box 5.10). When faced with delayed emergence, it is recommended that the anesthesiologist use a diagnostic algorithm to rule out pharmacologic, metabolic, and structural causes. The diagnostic approach must be sequential to maximize efficiency and prompt intervention. Begin with evaluating the residual effects of anesthetics and muscle relaxants followed by metabolic causes including infection, hyper/hypoglycemia, and electrolyte imbalances. Hypothermia and acid base disorders should be ruled out as well. Finally, imaging to assess intracranial pathology such as cerebral hemorrhage and stroke and consulting with neurology/neurosurgery would be indicated.

5.2.10. Rational opioid use

Intraoperative opioid administration blunts sympathetic and stress responses to laryngoscopy and surgical stimulation while preparing the patient for a smooth pain-free emergence. During the postoperative period, the rational use of opioid analgesia reduces the risk of collateral side effects such as respiratory depression and may

Box 5.10 Causes of delayed emergence from anesthesia

Pharmacological causes:
- Residual muscle relaxation
- Residual opioid or general anesthetic effect

Metabolic causes:
- Hypoglycemia or hyperglycemia
- Hypernatremia or hyponatremia
- Hypermagnesemia
- Hypothermia
- Drug intoxication (alcohol, central nervous system depressants)
- Metabolic encephalopathy (septic, hepatic, uremic)

Structural cerebral causes:
- Stroke
- Intracranial hemorrhage
- Seizures or post-ictal status

have an impact on length of stay and hospital costs. Knowledge of pharmacokinetic properties of different opioid medications is paramount to planning a sound perioperative analgesic plan. It is reasonable to use an intermediate acting agent like fentanyl during induction of anesthesia, whereas long-acting medications (e.g., hydromorphone, morphine) may be preferred in anticipation of emergence from anesthesia to provide pain relief in postanesthesia care. On the other hand, when rapid emergence is desirable, remifentanil infusions might be the first choice.

Intraoperative titration based on physiological variables such as heart rate and respiratory frequency is advisable. Special caution is recommended in patients with renal dysfunction.

Regardless of the opioid regimen chosen, the anesthesiologist must be vigilant against unwanted effects and monitor the patient accordingly. Finally, the administration of opioids as sole analgesic agent is an obsolete practice. A multimodal approach in which opioid agents represent one facet is better tolerated by patients and optimizes clinical effect while minimizing toxicity. This multimodal approach should include nonopioid drug administration and the use of regional anesthetic techniques.

5.2.11. Intraoperative hypotension and hypertension

Hypotension results from a decrease in cardiac output, peripheral vascular resistance, or both. Decreases in cardiac output may be the consequence of insufficient preload or contractility or increased afterload and tachy/bradyarrhythmias, whereas peripheral vascular resistance is diminished due to vasodilation. During anesthesia, the variables governing the maintenance of mean arterial pressure are affected by the administered medications, surgical bleeding and trauma, and physiologic changes associated with stress. It is difficult to isolate a single factor responsible for an episode of intraoperative hypotension; however, application of a systematic diagnostic algorithm helps the anesthesiologist to identify the most common correctable causes and to intervene in a timely fashion. Checking monitor variables and performing a quick physical exam should lead to a sound evaluation of a possible differential diagnosis. Treatment should be cause-specific; however, administration of fluid boluses and vasopressors as intermediate or final therapy are nearly universal, acknowledging the virtues and contraindications of each medication.

Hypertension during the intraoperative period is common in both pediatric and adult cases. The consequences of hypertensive episodes are deleterious and include cardiac ischemic events, intracranial hemorrhage, and stroke. Although rapid treatment is indicated, two factors must be taken into account before instituting therapy: identification of primary cause and negative effects of exaggerated correction of blood pressure. Common causes of hypertension are listed in Table 5.5. Ideally, blood pressure should

Table 5.5. Intraoperative causes of hypotension and hypertension

Hypotension	Hypertension
Hypovolemia/bleeding	Light anesthesia
Pharmacologically induced vasodilatation	Hypoxemia
Pneumothorax	Hypercapnia
Pulmonary embolism (thrombotic or venous air)	Hypothermia
Cardiac tamponade Myocardial ischemia	Hypoglycemia
Anaphylactic reaction	Malignant hyperthermia
Sepsis	Thyroid crisis
Inferior vena cava compression (pneumoperitoneum or manual compression)	Unrecognized cocaine/amphetamine intoxication
Monitor artifact	Intracranial hypertension

be maintained within 20% of baseline ranges, to avoid risk of end-organ hypoperfusion. When more pronounced decreases of blood pressure occur, rapid treatment and monitoring of signs of end-organ damage are indicated.

Further Reading

Akinci SB, Kanbak M, Guler A, Aypar U. Remifentanil versus fentanyl for short-term analgesia-based sedation in mechanically ventilated postoperative children. *Paediatr Anaesth*. 2005;15(10):870–878.

American Society of Anesthesiologists. Continuum of depth of sedation: definition of general anesthesia and levels of sedation/analgesia. Committee of Origin: Quality Management and Departmental Administration; approved by the ASA House of Delegates on October 13, 1999; last amended on October 15, 2014.

Cole DJ, Domino KB. Depth of anesthesia. In: Murray MJ, Harrison BA, Mueller JT, Rose SH, Wass CT, Wedel DJ, eds. *Faust's Anesthesiology Review*, 4th ed. Philadelphia: Elsevier; 2014; ch 18, pp 38–40.

Ehrenfeld JM, Funk LM, Van Schalkwyk J, Merry AF, Sandberg WS, Gawande A. The incidence of hypoxemia during surgery: evidence from two institutions. *Can J Anaesth*. 2010 Oct;57(10):888–897.

Elmquist L. Decision making for extubation of the post-anesthetic patient. *Crit Care Nurs Q*. 1992;15(1):82–86.

Gan TJ, Meyer T, Apfel CC, et al. Department of Anesthesiology, Duke University Medical Center. Consensus guidelines for managing postoperative nausea and vomiting. *Anesth Analg*. 2003;97(1):62–71.

Gandhi K, Baratta JL, Heitz JW, Schwenk ES, Vaghari B, Viscusi ER. Acute pain management in the postanesthesia care unit. *Anesthesiol Clin*. 2012;30(3):e1–15.

Joosten A, Alexander B, Delaporte A, Lilot M, Rinehart J, Cannesson M. Perioperative goal directed therapy using automated closed-loop fluid management: the future? *Anaesthesiol Intensive Ther*. 2015;47(5):517–523.

Joosten A, Rinehart J, Cannesson M. Perioperative goal directed therapy: evidence and compliance are two sides of the same coin. *Rev Esp Anestesiol Reanim*. 2015;62(4):181–183.

Lee JW. Fluid and electrolyte disturbances in critically ill patients. *Electrolyte Blood Press*. 2010;8(2):72–81.

Marik PE, Varon J. Perioperative hypertension: a review of current and emerging therapeutic agents. *J Clin Anesth*. 2009;21(3):220–229.

Mastronardi P, Cafiero T. Rational use of opioids. *Minerva Anestesiol*. 2001;67(4):332.

McNarry AF, Patel A. The evolution of airway management—new concepts and conflicts with traditional practice. *Br J Anaesth*. 2017;119(Suppl. 1):i154–i166.

Misal US, Joshi SA, Shaikh MM. Delayed recovery from anesthesia: a postgraduate educational review. *Anesth Essays Res*. 2016;10(2):164–172.

Navarro LH, Bloomstone JA, Auler JO Jr, et al. Perioperative fluid therapy: a statement from the international Fluid Optimization Group. *Perioper Med.* 2015;4:3.

Nunes RR, Porto VC, Miranda VT, de Andrade NQ, Carneiro LM. Risk factor for intraoperative awareness. *Rev Bras Anestesiol.* 2012;62(3):365–374.

Sloan TB, Jameson L, Janik D. Evoked potentials. In: Cotrell JE, Young WL, eds. *Cotrell and Young's Neuroanesthesia*, 6th ed. Philadelphia: Mosby Elsevier; 2017; ch 6, pp 114–126.

Spahn DR, Moch H, Hofmann A, Isbister JP. Patient blood management: the pragmatic solution for the problems with blood transfusions. *Anesthesiology.* 2008;109(6):951–953.

Universal Protocol for Preventing Wrong Site, Wrong Procedure, and Wrong Person Surgery. Guidance for health care professionals. Joint Commission. Rockville, MD: Agency for Healthcare Research and Quality.

Vulser H, Airagnes G, Lahlou-Laforêt K, et al. Psychiatric consequences of intraoperative awareness: short review and case series. *Gen Hosp Psychiatry.* 2015;37(1):94–95.

World Alliance for Patient Safety. *Implementation Manual Surgical Safety Checklist*, 1st ed. Geneva: World Health Organization.

Chapter 6

Crisis Management in the Perioperative Setting

Claudia F. Clavijo, Ronnie Zeidan,
and Efrain Riveros-Perez

6.1. Laryngospasm and aspiration of gastric contents

6.1.1. Laryngospasm

Laryngospasm is a forceful and sustained spasm of the laryngeal muscles resulting in partial or complete loss of the airway. Even though laryngospasm can occur in the conscious patient, it is most common during emergence or in patients who are in a light plane of anesthesia. It is recommended that extubation be performed either deeply anesthetized with patient breathing spontaneously (stage 3) or in an awake patient (Table 6.1).

Presentation Laryngospasm is more common in pediatric than in adult patients. Periglottic secretions or foreign bodies such as the endotracheal tube can cause sensory stimulation of the superior laryngeal nerve. This protective mechanism closes the glottis opening by constricting the laryngeal muscles (by vocal cord adduction alone or in conjunction with adduction of false vocal cords) to avoid pulmonary aspiration. Complete or partial closure of the airway opening prevents airflow during the inspiratory effort, compromising oxygenation and ventilation. The large negative intrathoracic pressure generated during laryngospasm can produce negative pressure pulmonary edema.

Table 6.1. Depth of anesthesia	
Stage 1	Analgesia
Stage 2	Excitement
Stage 3	Surgical anesthesia
Stage 4	Medullary paralysis

Immediate management

- Early recognition and treatment are essential to avoid significant morbidity.
- The first step is to open the oropharynx and clear secretions.
- Apply continuous positive airway pressure with 100% oxygen concentration.
- Administer intravenous (IV) lidocaine 1–1.5 mg/kg (evidence is conflicting).
- If laryngospasm persists, administer succinylcholine 0.25–1 mg/kg.
- When laryngospasm occurs during a light plane of anesthesia, deepening of anesthesia by providing a bolus of propofol or increasing the concentration of inhalational agent is recommended.

6.1.2. Perioperative pulmonary aspiration

Also known as Mendelson's syndrome, pulmonary aspiration is the inhalation of gastric, oro-, or naso-pharyngeal content into the respiratory tract. This material could be solid or particulate, acid gastric fluid, or even blood. Evaluating the risk of aspiration and modifying the anesthesia plan accordingly is imperative to reduce aspiration and related morbidity. Although the incidence of perioperative aspiration is approximately 1:3,000, 25% of patients who aspirate develop significant respiratory morbidity and mortality with an even higher incidence in the elderly and in patients who are classified as ASA physical classification III or greater.

Presentation. Aspiration can happen at any time, even before induction, but is more common during intubation and extubation of the trachea. Intraoperatively, regurgitation occurs more often than active vomiting. A common factor is an attempt to intubate a patient who is not completely paralyzed. Laryngoscopy and intubation can activate a gag reflex and vomiting. Extubation in a weak or not fully conscious patient offers the same risk. Aspiration of particulate material can cause obstruction of the airway, interfere with ventilation and oxygenation, and consequently produce hypoxia. Aspiration of acid gastric contents could cause progressive dyspnea, hypoxia and pneumonitis, aspiration pneumonia, and acute respiratory distress syndrome. Acidity and the volume of the aspirated material determine the severity of the syndrome and its associated mortality. Fasting time should always be reviewed and confirmed with patients before anesthesia starts to ensure adequate nothing per mouth status in elective cases. Patients who are sicker and present for emergent procedures are at higher risk of aspiration, particularly those who have eaten recently or have a small bowel obstruction or ileus.

Pathophysiology. The protective laryngeal reflexes (coughing, expiration, and laryngospasm), the gastroesophageal junction, and the upper esophageal sphincter provide a physiologic protective mechanism to decrease aspiration risk. During induction, maintenance, and emergence, this protective mechanism is reduced. Inadequate depth of anesthesia, inadequate muscle relaxation, or surgical stimulation may induce gastrointestinal motor responses and increase gastric pressure above the pressure of the lower esophageal sphincter. This enables gastric contents to move upward in the gastrointestinal tract and enter the respiratory tract. Although gastrointestinal stimulants, histamine-2 receptor antagonists, proton pump inhibitors, antacids, and antiemetics are known to decrease acidity and gastric volume, there is no evidence that they reduce aspiration risk. Patients considered at high risk of aspiration (Table 6.2) may benefit from these medications, but routine use is not recommended.

Immediate management

- Carefully suction aspirated material.
- If particulate material is seen, bronchoscopy should be performed.
- Support respiratory function.
- Targeted antibiotic therapy is used if aspiration pneumonia develops.

Lavage with saline has not proven to be useful; on the contrary, it can increase the spread of aspirate. Prophylactic antibiotics and steroids are ineffective in preventing pneumonia or lung inflammation or in improving outcomes.

6.2. Oxygen failure in the OR

The institution's medical gas pipeline is the primary source of oxygen and medical gases for the anesthesia machine. Unfortunately, there may be problems with this source, including high or inadequate pressure, contamination, or failure of the structural equipment due to external sources. An oxygen failure can be caused by crossover or inadequate pressure. Crossover, the erroneous switch between oxygen and another gas (e.g., nitrous oxide), has almost been eliminated in the United States thanks to the implementation of the Diameter-Index Safety System, a color-coded and size-shape specific outlet system that prevents wrong gas connections. Inadequate pressure results in insufficient oxygenation of a patient under general anesthesia.

Oxygen failure in the operating room (OR) is an uncommon but potentially catastrophic incident. Anesthesia providers have an important role in keeping patients safe during such an event.

Table 6.2. Risk factors associated with aspiration

Patient factors	
Full stomach	Emergency surgery
	Inadequate fasting time
	Gastrointestinal obstruction
Delayed gastric emptying	Systemic disease (diabetes mellitus, chronic kidney disease)
	Recent trauma
	Opioids
	Elevated intracranial pressure
	Previous gastrointestinal surgery
	Pregnancy (including active labor)
Incompetent lower esophageal sphincter	Hiatal hernia
	Recurrent regurgitation
	Dyspepsia
	Previous upper gastrointestinal surgery
	Pregnancy
Esophageal disease	Previous gastrointestinal surgery
	Morbid obesity
Surgical factors	Upper gastrointestinal surgery
	Lithotomy or head down position
	Laparoscopy
	Cholecystectomy
Anesthetic factors	Light anesthesia
	Positive pressure ventilation
	Supraglottic airway devices
	Length of surgery > 2 h
	Difficult airway
Device factors	First generation supraglottic airway devices

Adapted from the *British Journal of Anaesthesia*.

Presentation The hospital pipeline is the primary source of all gases and the pressure within the pipelines is 50 PSI which is the normal working pressure of the anesthesia delivery system. The loss of oxygen resulting in a pressure below 30 PSI will activate an audible and visible alert in the anesthesia machine. Modern

> **Box 6.1 Immediate management**
>
> - Determine whether oxygen failure is the source of the alert and call for help.
> - Open the backup oxygen cylinder fully. This will re-pressurize the anesthesia machine.
> - Disconnect pipeline oxygen.
> - Manually ventilate using the breathing circuit on the machine.
> - Reduce flow to the safe minimum to match patient oxygen consumption.
> - Continue to administer inhalational agent.
> - Ensure that patient is being ventilated with 100% oxygen concentration by using a gas analyzer.

anesthesia equipment will also shut off the flow of other gases if oxygen pressure falls below 20 PSI to avoid hypoxic gas mixtures (Box 6.1).

If this strategy fails to pressurize the anesthesia machine:

- Connect the patient to a self-inflating bag with positive pressure capabilities.
- Connect the self-inflating bag device to the oxygen tank on the back of the anesthesia machine and ventilate the patient.
- If the oxygen tank on the back of the anesthesia machine does not work, call for a portable oxygen tank to connect the self-inflating device and ventilate the patient.
- Prepare to transition to total IV anesthesia to maintain anesthesia in case the oxygen failure is caused by power failure and the inhalation agent cannot be delivered.

Note the importance of checking the backup oxygen cylinder pressure as part of the daily anesthesia machine check.

6.3. Anaphylaxis

Anaphylactic reactions are sudden and exaggerated responses to an allergen. They are IgE-mediated type 1 immune reactions that produce mast cell and basophil degranulation as well as activation of vasoactive mediators. Anaphylactic reactions affect all organ systems and can produce a life-threatening response due to cardiovascular shock and acute respiratory failure. The incidence of anaphylactic reactions during anesthesia has been reported to be 1:5,000 to 1:25,000. Antibiotics (penicillin and cephalosporins) are the most common source of anaphylactic reactions in surgical patients. Latex is another important allergen in the perioperative period.

Anaphylactoid reactions have the same clinical presentation, but they are not mediated by an IgE antibody-antigen interaction. These types of reactions are the result of direct nonimmune–mediated stimulation, by medications or other substances, on mast cells and or basophils producing histamine release. Even though anaphylactic reactions to anesthetic medications are rare, and anaphylactoid reactions are reported more frequently, true anaphylactic reactions have been reported in particular with the use of muscle relaxants, even without previous exposure. The proposed mechanism seems to be a cross-reaction with food, prescription medications, and over-the-counter medications that share tertiary or quaternary ion epitopes with muscle relaxants. The incidence of anaphylaxis to propofol is approximately 1:60,000. Adverse reactions to opioids are usually nonimmune histamine release, while reported reactions to local anesthetics are due to local anesthetic toxic or vasovagal responses or are related to epinephrine toxicity. Allergic reactions to ketamine, etomidate, and benzodiazepines are extremely rare.

Presentation The most common signs and symptoms are seen in the cardiac, respiratory, and cutaneous systems. After exposure to an allergen, the patient presents with a sudden cough, dyspnea, bronchospasm, wheezing, increased in-peak inspiratory pressure, laryngeal and pulmonary edema, and hypoxia. $ETCO_2$ and SaO_2 decrease simultaneously. The airway can be lost easily if the anaphylactic reaction is not promptly treated. Hypotension, tachycardia or bradycardia, arrhythmias, and arrest are also seen. Early cutaneous manifestations include erythema, flushing, pruritus, facial edema, and urticaria. Disseminated intravascular coagulation (DIC) and renal failure are also possible in severe cases. Keep in mind that some signs may not be present in anesthetized patients.

Pathophysiology Previous sensitization or cross-sensitization are necessary for an anaphylactic reaction to occur. Two IgE molecules (antigen-antibody reaction) initiate degranulation of mast cells and basophils and activate the release of vasoactive mediators (histamine, tryptase, prostaglandins, leukotrines, and proteoglycans). Prior sensitization is not required to start anaphylactoid reactions.

Histamine and leukotriene production leads to vasodilation and increased vascular permeability. Prostaglandins and proteases such as tryptase produce broncoconstriction. Proteoglycans activate a coagulation cascade and can trigger DIC. Box 6.2 details the immediate management of anaphylaxis.

Box 6.2 Immediate management

- Discontinue possible allergen (medications, latex products, blood, colloids, etc.).
- Ensure maintenance of the airway; consider early intubation or tracheostomy.
- Administer 100% oxygen.
- Discontinue volatile anesthetics if hypotension is present.
- Administer 1 to 2 L of lactated Ringer's.
- Dilute and administer epinephrine. Dose and route of administration will depend on severity of reaction (0.01–0.5 mg IV or intramuscular).
- Infusion of epinephrine may be needed.
- If there is no IV access, consider intratracheal administration of epinephrine.
- Administer
  - beta-2-agonist (albuterol inhaler or terbutaline inhaled)
  - corticosteroid (hydrocortisone up to 200 mg IV or methylprednisolone 1–2 mg/kg)
  - antihistamines (diphenhydramine 50–75 mg IV)
  - vasopressin (2–4 units IV)
- Consider additional IV access and invasive blood pressure monitoring.

75

6.4. Local anesthetic systemic toxicity

Local anesthetics are ubiquitous agents in clinical practice. They are administered for topical absorption through skin and mucosal surfaces, local infiltration, peripheral nerve blocks, and neuraxial techniques and as an IV infusion. Local anesthetics are part of the pharmacological armamentarium in diverse contexts including dental practice, emergency rooms, general wards, and ORs. Awareness of local anesthetic systemic toxicity (LAST) is sometimes limited due to the wrong belief that these medications lack significant side effects.

Pathophysiology Some pharmacokinetic and pharmacodynamic properties of local anesthetics determine both their clinical effects and toxicity profile. The degree of ionization (determined by the compound pKa) determines the ability to cross lipid membranes and the time of onset, whereas lipophilicity is associated with potency and protein binding with duration of action. Affinity of local

Box 6.3 Local anesthetic systemic toxicity clinical presentation

Central nervous system:
- Perioral numbness
- Metallic taste
- Anxiety and confusion
- Visual changes
- Muscle twitches
- Seizures
- Coma and respiratory depression

Cardiovascular system:
- Tachycardia
- Hypertension
- Bradycardia
- Hypotension
- Arrhythmias
- Asystole

anesthetics to the protein domain of the voltage-activated rapid sodium channels in excitable tissue is the main mechanism of action of local anesthetic agents. Although all local anesthetics can cause LAST, there are differences in neurologic and cardiac toxicity among different agents. As a rule of thumb, the potency of the medication parallels its toxicity profile, so that bupivacaine is more cardiotoxic than lidocaine.

Clinical presentation. Typically, clinical presentation of LAST starts with signs and symptoms of central nervous system (CNS) excitation followed by CNS inhibition, cardiac excitatory signs, and eventually cardiac arrest. However, in some cases, this sequence is not present, and cardiac toxicity can occur without prior warning signs (Box 6.3).

Prevention and management. The risk of developing LAST depends on patient factors (Box 6.4), site of administration of the agent, and the administered dose. Therapeutic dose range recommendations for every local anesthetic must be followed, recognizing that for highly liposoluble local anesthetics, the addition of epinephrine does not change the toxic dose.

Vascular supply surrounding the site of administration determines systemic absorption and the risk of LAST. In order of decreasing risk, intercostal, caudal, epidural, interfascial plane, psoas, sciatic, cervical, and brachial plexus blocks carry some risk of LAST. Use of ultrasound guidance for peripheral blocks reduces the risk of vascular absorption of the anesthetic. Slow dosing techniques

- Extremes of age
- Limited physiologic reserve (cardiac, hepatic, renal)
- Pregnancy
- Metabolic disturbances (acidosis, hypoxia, electrolyte abnormalities)
- Carnitine deficiency

preceded by aspiration are advised in order to limit a rapid plasma concentration rise and to allow time to detect toxic manifestations of an unintentional intravascular injection.

The approach to management of LAST must include different simultaneous and sequential actions in accordance with published guidelines. The pillars of successful management of these cases are early recognition, rapid response, maintenance of airway patency and breathing, seizure suppression, and cardiovascular support (Box 6.5).

Box 6.5 Management of LAST

Stop injection.

Get help.

Manage airway:
- 100% oxygen
- Assist or control ventilation as indicated
- Airway instrumentation as indicated

Seizure treatment:
- Benzodiazepines (midazolam)
- Caution with propofol if hemodynamic instability is present

Contact personnel or facility to set up cardiopulmonary bypass.

Cardiovascular support and arrhythmia treatment:
- Basic and advanced cardiac life support
- Reduce epinephrine dose to less than 1 mg

Lipid emulsion (20%) therapy:
- Bolus 1.5 mL/kg in 10 min
- 0.25 mL/kg/min infusion
- Double infusion to 0.5 mL/kg/min if still hypotensive
- Repeat bolus for cardiovascular collapse
- Recommended upper limit of 10 mL/kg over the first 30 minutes

Transfer patient to a monitored setting.

6.5. Malignant hyperthermia

Malignant hyperthermia (MH) is a hypermetabolic condition that occurs secondary to administration of definite triggering anesthetic agents. Patients susceptible to MH have genetic alterations of muscular receptors involved in sarcoplasmic calcium dynamics, resulting in massive contraction, anaerobic metabolism and muscle fiber breakdown, when the patient is exposed to certain anesthetic medications (Box 6.6).

Pathophysiology. The typical sequence consists of an increase in sarcoplasmic calcium, followed by severe generalized muscle contractions that lead to a massive production of carbon dioxide, followed by accelerated lactate production and muscle breakdown. The landmark signs resulting from the cascade are hyperthermia, muscle rigidity, respiratory and metabolic acidosis, myoglobinuria, and hyperkalemia.

Clinical presentation. Clinical presentation starts with unexplained tachycardia, hypercapnia (increased end-tidal CO_2), and masseter or generalized muscle rigidity. Hyperthermia is rarely an early sign. When the patient is under anesthesia, the first sign is an elevation in end-tidal CO_2, whereas muscle rigidity might be the first sign when the syndrome presents during the postoperative period. When MH is suspected, evaluation of acid-base status, serum potassium, serum creatine kinase, and urinary myoglobin are indicated (Box 6.7).

Management. When the anesthesiologist suspects MH, treatment of a presumed case should start. An appropriately stocked MH cart should be moved to the OR and additional personnel notified. Dantrolene must be reconstituted and administered as per guidelines. Additional assistance can be obtained from the Malignant Hyperthermia Association of the United States hotline (1-800-644-9737). Treatment strategies can be classified into supportive, therapy for complications, and therapies directly targeting MH (Box 6.8).

Box 6.6 Nonsafe anesthetic medications in malignant hyperthermia–susceptible individuals (triggering agents)
• Succinylcholine
• Isoflurane
• Desflurane
• Isoflurane
• Enflurane
• Halothane

Box 6.7 Differential diagnosis of malignant hyperthermia

- Insufficient anesthetic/analgesic level
- Hypoventilation
- Equipment failure
- Artificial overheating
- Transfusion reaction
- Drug intoxication (cocaine, amphetamines)
- Alcohol withdrawal
- Neuroleptic malignant syndrome
- Sepsis
- Thyroid storm
- Undiagnosed pheochromocytoma

After finishing the surgical procedure, the patient should be transferred to the intensive care unit, where supportive measures and monitoring must continue. A significant number of patients have recurrence of MH signs during the postoperative period. Dantrolene can be stopped when body temperature returns to

Box 6.8 Treatment of malignant hyperthermia

Supportive therapy:

- Optimize oxygenation (FiO_2 100%).
- Monitor ventilation and adjust according to arterial blood gases.
- Monitor hemodynamic status (adequate vascular access).

Therapy directed to MH:

- Discontinue any triggering agents.
- Change anesthesia machine (halogenated-naïve).
- Start total intravenous anesthesia.
- Administer dantrolene.

  Loading bolus 2.5 mg/kg IV

  Subsequent bolus doses of 1 mg/kg until MH signs abate

Therapy for complications:

- Monitor and treat acidosis.
- Monitor and treat hyperkalemia.

(Continued)

Box 6.8 Continued

- Treat cardiac arrhythmias according to etiology and hemodynamic status.
- Monitor temperature and start cooling maneuvers as necessary.
- Monitor creatine kinase levels.
- Treat myoglobinuria (hydration, diuretics, bicarbonate).
- Monitor for disseminated intravascular coagulation.

normal, muscle rigidity subsides, creatine kinase levels are trending down, there is no evidence of myoglobinuria, and the metabolic status is normal.

Finally, it is important that all anesthesia providers are aware of the location of the MH cart and that the hospital pharmacy has a protocol in place for periodic check of its contents and expiration dates (Box 6.9). Orientation materials regarding immediate response guidelines in case of MH should be provided during orientation of anesthesia providers and nursing staff working in the OR.

6.6. ACLS for cardiac arrest in the OR

In the United States, an estimated 350,000 to 400,000 sudden cardiac arrests occur outside the hospital setting. Although cardiac arrests are fairly common in the United States, perioperative

Box 6.9 Malignant hyperthermia cart contents

- Dantrolene
  - Dantrum®/Revonto® (contain mannitol) 36 vials
  - Ryanodex® 3 vials
- Sterile water for injection
- Sodium bicarbonate
- Dextrose 50%
- Calcium chloride
- Regular insulin
- Lidocaine for injection (2%)
- Refrigerated cold saline

cardiac arrests are relatively rare. ACLS protocols were originally developed to aid first responders in resuscitating individuals found unresponsive in the community. Although the most common causes of cardiac arrests in the community differ from the most common causes of acute cardiac arrests in the perioperative setting, the fundamental principles of ACLS can be applied to situations in the OR (see Table 6.3 and Figure 6.1).

Cardiac arrest during anesthesia is unique because it is usually witnessed and anticipated. The patient's medical history should be known by the anesthesiologist, allowing him or her to support the patient's physiological state which allows for rapid initiation of ACLS. In a review of cardiac arrests associated with anesthesia, the most common electrocardiogram rhythms at the time of arrest were bradycardia (23%); asystole (22%); tachydysrhythmia, including ventricular tachycardia and ventricular fibrillation (14%); and normal rhythm (7%).

A stepwise therapeutic approach to cardiac arrest in the OR based on the 2010 American Heart Association ACLS sequence and the International Liaison Committee on Resuscitation consensus statement on postcardiac arrest syndrome should be considered in directing therapy in the OR (Box 6.10).

Table 6.3. Common causes of acute cardiac arrests in the perioperative setting		
Cardiovascular	Anesthetic	Respiratory
Vasovagal	IV anesthetic overdose	Hypoxemia
Hypovolemic shock	Inhalation anesthetic overdose	Auto-PEEP
Gas embolism	Neuroaxial anesthetic with a high level of sympathectomy	Acute bronchospasm
Acute electrolyte imbalance	Local anesthetic toxicity	
Transfusion reaction	Malignant hyperthermia	
Anaphylaxis		
Acute coronary syndrome		
Tension pneumothorax		
Oculocardiac reflex		
Pacemaker failure		

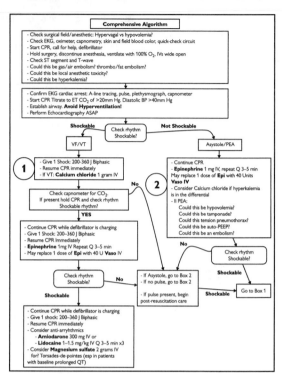

Figure 6.1. Comprehensive algorithm

Box 6.10 Corrective measures for clinical progression to shock

- Recognize a true crisis.
- Call for help.
- Call for defibrillator.
- Hold surgery and anesthetic if feasible.
- Administer FIO$_2$ of 1.0.
- Confirm airway positioning and functioning.
- Assess oxygen source and anesthetic circuit integrity.
- Review ETCO$_2$ trends before hemodynamic instability.

Generate a differential diagnosis:

- Evaluate procedure and consult with procedural colleagues.
- Review recently administered medications.

Box 6.10 Continued

- Obtain chest radiograph to rule out tension pneumothorax if airway resistance acutely increased.
- Obtain echocardiogram (transesophageal echocardiogram if patient's trachea is intubated or if patient has a surgically prepped chest) to evaluate ventricular filling, ventricular function, and valvular function and to exclude pericardial tamponade (Focused Echocardiographic Evaluation and Resuscitation exam).
- Empiric replacement therapy with corticosteroids (in patients who have not been previously treated with steroids, hydrocortisone 50 mg IV and fludrocortisone 50 μg PO/nasogastric).

Cardiac arrest in the perioperative setting is thankfully a rare event which can be a result of a unique and diverse spectrum of causes (Table 6.4). Anesthesiologists must have a thorough understanding of the ACLS algorithm to be facile in the adaptation of the ACLS algorithm to treat cardiac arrests in the OR. Since it is both uncommon and heterogeneous, perioperative cardiac arrest has

Table 6.4. Perioperative cardiac arrest	
Circulation	o Check pulse for 10 sec
	o Effective two-rescuer CPR:
	1. Minimize interruptions
	2. Chest compression rate 100 compressions·min⁻¹
	3. Depth 2 in, full decompression, real-time feedback.
	4. Titrate CPR to A-line BP diastolic 40 mmHg or ETCO₂ 20 mmHg
	o Drug reaction
	o Attempt CVL placement
Airway	o Bag mask ventilation until intubation
	o Endotracheal intubation
	o Difficult airway algorithm
Breathing	o Respiratory rate 10 breaths·min⁻¹
	o VT to visible chest rise
	o T₁ 1 sec
	o Consider inspiratory threshold valve (ITV)

(Continued)

Table 6.4. Continued	
Defibrillation	o Defibrillation if shockable rhythm
	o Repeat defibrillation every 2 min if shockable rhythm
Postcardiac arrest	o Invasive monitoring
	o Final surgical anesthetic plan

ACLS = advanced cardiac life support; BLS = basic life support;
CPR = cardiopulmonary resuscitation; FIO2 = fraction of inspired oxygen
concentration; ETCO2 = end-tidal carbon dioxide; BP = blood pressure;
CVL = central venous line; VT = tidal volume; TI = inspiratory time; ICU = intensive
care unit.

not been described or studied to the same extent as cardiac arrest in the community; thus, recommendations for management must be predicated on expert opinion and physiological understanding rather than on the standards currently being used in the generation of ACLS protocols in the community.

6.7. Surgical site infections

Surgical site infections (SSI), defined as occurring within 30 days of surgery or within 90 days if a prosthetic implant is utilized, are the second most common cause of nosocomial infections.

SSIs are believed to affect 500,000 patients annually and can lead to a two- to 11-fold increased risk of death compared to operative patients without an SSI. SSIs contribute to an increased hospital length of stay, a reduced quality of life, and death. From a cost perspective, SSIs are believed to account for up to $7 billion annually in health care expenditures. It is estimated that 40% to 60% of SSIs are preventable. Given the widespread implications of SSIs on the health care system, US regulatory agencies (including Medicare) will no longer reimburse institutions for certain SSIs.

The goal of perioperative antimicrobial prophylaxis is to obtain blood and tissue drug levels that exceed the minimum inhibitory concentration for the organisms that are most likely to be encountered prior to surgical incision. Ideally an antibiotic administration should be completed before incision, but Centers for Medicare and Medicaid Services guidelines consider starting an infusion before incision for those antibiotics that require slow administration before incision adequate. When possible, for drugs requiring a slow (>30 min) infusion, the infusion should be initiated preoperatively. For surgical procedures in which a tourniquet is used, the entirety of the recommended dose should be completed at least five minutes prior to tourniquet inflation.

The selection of drug choice is imperative in accurately mounting a defense against organisms that most commonly cause SSIs.

When deciding on antibiotic prophylaxis, dose and timing should be determined by a hospital committee based on national guidelines. A commonly utilized drug of choice for prophylaxis for a multitude of surgical procedures, which do not violate the chronically colonized organs, is cefazolin, due to its antimicrobial properties against streptococcus, methicillin-susceptible staphylococci, and some Gram-negative bacteria. These microbes commonly colonize skin flora and cefazolin (first-generation cephalosporin) adequately covers these organisms.

As anesthesiologists, it is imperative to communicate with the surgical team and confirm selection of antibiotics either during the time-out or before that event. Effective communication is imperative because antibiotics may not be indicated or may be held until after surgical culture is isolated. Communication also serves as an additional safety mechanism in the event that a patient has an allergy to specific classes of antibiotics. Many patients report an allergy to penicillin. It should be noted that penicillin allergy is almost never a contraindication to cefazolin or other cephalosporins unless there is a documented history of anaphylaxis or other serious reactions. A thorough preoperative discussion with a patient is vital in determining the reaction a patient has had, in order to avoid choosing an antimicrobial with reduced efficacy, increased cost, and a higher risk of side effects.

The risk of infective endocarditis (IE) should be given special consideration in specific patient populations undergoing certain types of procedures. The American Heart Association no longer recommends prophylaxis solely to prevent IE from genitourinary and gastrointestinal procedures. IE prophylaxis is recommended for dental procedures for patients with cardiac lesions with the highest risk of adverse outcomes from IE.

Patients with a high risk of IE in which prophylaxis is indicated include those who have

- a prosthetic cardiac valve or prosthetic material used for cardiac valve repair
- Previous IE
- Congenital heart disease (CHD)
  - Unrepaired cyanotic congenital heart disease, including palliative shunts and conduits
  - Completely repaired congenital heart defect with prosthetic material or device, whether placed by surgery or catheter intervention, during the first six months after procedure
  - Repaired CHD with residual defects at the site or adjacent to the site of a prosthetic patch or prosthetic device
  - Cardiac transplant recipients who develop cardiac valvulopathy

85

6.8. OR fires

According to the American Society of Anesthesiologists (ASA), of the more than 28 million surgeries performed each year in the United States, anywhere from 50 to 200 may experience a fire in the OR. OR fires can potentially be lethal or cause serious harm to patients and providers. For the purpose of this discussion we define surgical airway fires and OR fires based on ASA's 2013 "Practice Advisory for the Prevention and Management of Operating Room Fires." OR fires occur on or near patients who are under anesthesia care, including surgical fires, airway fires, and fires within the airway circuit. A surgical fire is defined as a fire that occurs on or in a patient. An airway fire is a specific type of surgical fire that occurs in a patient's airway (which may or may not include fire that in the attached breathing circuit).

Elements which compose OR fires are routinely referred to as the "fire triad." This triad is composed of an oxidizer, an ignition source, and fuel. To effectively prevent OR fires, successful removal of one of these elements of the triad is required (Table 6.5).

The most common oxidizers encountered in an OR are oxygen and nitrous oxide. An oxidizer-enriched atmosphere occurs when there is any increase in oxygen concentration above room air level and or the presence of any concentration of nitrous oxide. The

Table 6.5. Components of the "fire triad"

Oxidizers	Ignition source	Fuel
Oxygen (O_2)	Patient	Malfunctioning electrical devices
Nitrous oxide (N_2O)	Drapes	Electrosurgical devices
	Blankets	Electrocautery devices
	Gauze	Lasers
	Sponges	Fiberoptic scopes
	Dressings	Defibrillators
	Alcohol containing solutions	
	O_2 masks	
	Ventilator	
	Tracheal tubes	

oxidizer-enriched atmosphere in an OR commonly occurs within a closed or semiclosed breathing system.

General OR fire prevention strategies involve minimizing or completely avoiding oxidizer-enriched atmospheres, fuels, and ignition. Identifying high-risk procedures is paramount in preventing OR fires. A high-risk procedure in this context is defined as one in which an ignition source can come in proximity to an oxidizer-enriched atmosphere and includes tonsillectomy, tracheostomy, removal of laryngeal papilloma, eye surgery, burr hole surgery, or any removal of lesions on the head, neck, or face. Some strategies to effectively reduce the risk of fires are minimizing the oxygen concentration to as low as possible, using a cuffed endotracheal tube to lessen the leak of oxygen, and utilizing a laser-resistant tracheal tube for laser procedures and a filling cuff with colored saline to allow for detection of a perforation. See the 2013 ASA Operating Room Fires Algorithm for more information.

Further Reading

Anderson WR, Brock-Utne JG. Oxygen pipeline supply failure: a coping strategy. *J Clin Monit.* 1991;7(1):39–41.

Bratzler DW, Dellinger EP, Olsen KM, Perl TM, Auwaerter PG, Bolon MK, Steinberg JP. Clinical practice guidelines for antimicrobial prophylaxis in surgery. *Surg Infec.* 2013:14(1):73–156.

Dewatcher P, Mouton-Faivre C, Emala C. Anaphylaxis and anesthesia: controversies and new insights. *Anesthesiology.* 2009;111:1141–1150.

Gavel G, Walker RWM. Laryngospasm in anaesthesia. Continuing Education in Anaesthesia. *Crit Care Pain.* 2014;14(2):47–51.

Hoegberg LC, Bania TC, Lavergne V, et al. Lipid Emulsion Workgroup. Systematic review of the effect of intravenous lipid emulsion therapy for local anesthetic toxicity. *Clin Toxicol.* 2016;54(3):167–193.

Larach MG, Gronert GA, Allen GC, Brandom BW, Lehman EB. Clinical presentation, treatment, and complications of malignant hyperthermia in North America from 1987 to 2006. *Anesth Analg.* 2010;110(2):498–507.

Litman RS, Flood CD, Kaplan RF, Kim YL, Tobin JR. Postoperative malignant hyperthermia: an analysis of cases from the North American Malignant Hyperthermia Registry. *Anesthesiology.* 2008;109(5):825–829.

Meeks DW, Lally KP, Carrick MM, Lew DF, Thomas EJ, Doyle PD, Kao LS. Compliance with guidelines to prevent surgical site infections: as simple as 1-2-3? *Am J Surg.* 2011;201(1):76–83.

Moitra VK, Gabrielli A, Maccioli GA, O'Connor MF. Anesthesia advanced circulatory life support. *Can J Anaesth.* 2012;59(6):586–603.

Practice guidelines for preoperative fasting and the use of pharmacologic agents to reduce the risk of pulmonary aspiration: application to healthy patients undergoing elective procedures. An update report by the American Society of Anesthesiologists Task Force on Preoperative

Fasting and the Use of Pharmacologic Agents to Reduce the Risk of Pulmonary Aspiration. *Anesthesiology*. 2017;126:376–393.

Runciman WB, Morris RW, Watterson LM, Williamson JA, Paix AD. Crisis management during anaesthesia: cardiac arrest. *Qual Saf Health Care*. 2005;14:e14.

Schumacher SD, Brockwell RC, Andrews JJ, Ogles D. Bulk liquid oxygen supply failure. *Anesthesiology*. 2004;100(1):186–189.

Shoham AB, Murray MJ. Perioperative pulmonary aspiration. In: Murray MJ, Harrison BA, Mueller JT, Rose SH, Wass CT, Wedel DJ, eds. *Faust's Anesthesiology Review*, 4th ed. Philadelphia: Elsevier; 2014 pp 570–571.

Wolfe JW, Butterworth JF. Local anesthetic systemic toxicity: update on mechanisms and treatment. *Curr Opin Anaesthesiol*. 2011;24(5):561–566.

Chapter 7

Postanesthesia Care on the Day of Surgery

Lindsey Van Drunen and Sanjay Dwarakanath

7.1. Safe patient transport

For the anesthesiologist, care of the surgical patient extends beyond the operating room (OR) to the postanesthesia care unit (PACU). Ensuring the patient remains safe during transport is the initial step of postanesthetic care (see Box 7.1). Most patients will be provided with supplemental oxygen (O_2) during transport. Different levels of monitoring are required based on the status of the patient. For example, a healthy, American Society of Anesthesiologists class I patient who undergoes an uneventful anesthetic and is able to be safely extubated at the end of a procedure may solely require vigilance by the anesthesiologist during transport. This includes watching for continued respirations as evidenced by chest rise and fall or feeling for exhaled breaths. In addition, verbally communicating with the patient can confirm upper airway patency. On the other hand, an intensive care unit (ICU) patient requires continuous electrocardiogram, heart rate, blood pressure via cuff or arterial line, and pulse oximetry monitoring. If the patient remains intubated, the anesthesiologist or an assistant must maintain manual ventilation. Occasionally, an ICU ventilator may be required for transport in extremely sick patients. Safe patient transport also includes confirming readily available intravenous (IV) access in case of emergency. Patient position during transport depends on the clinical profile of the patient and type of surgery. The reverse Trendelenburg or back-up position facilitates better tidal volume and prevention of atelectasis. The Trendelenburg position enhances preload due to drainage of blood from the lower extremities. The lateral position, especially in pediatric patients, prevents aspiration while helping maintain airway patency. Upon arrival to the PACU or ICU, the patient's blood pressure, pulse, oxygen saturation, and electrocardiogram should be recorded.

Box 7.1 Key points to consider for safe patient transport

- Ensure presence of transport team based on hospital policy (surgeon, nurse, etc.); consider asking for an assistant for transport.
- Inform attending anesthesiologist prior to transport.
- Anticipate need for airway equipment and medications (vasopressors, inotropes, analgesics, sedation, etc.) for transport.
- Continually assess A (airway), B (breathing), and C (circulation) during transport.
- Consider using a transport monitor depending on the patient and nature of the surgery.

7.2. Hand-off reporting to next level of care

As the patient transitions from the OR to either the ICU or PACU, a hand-off will occur between the anesthesia team and the care team, which will resume care of the patient postoperatively. The PACU care team usually involves a nurse and anesthesiology resident or attending. Typically, hand-offs include the medical history of the patient, operation, type of anesthesia, IV access, medications given, fluids administered, and estimated blood loss as well as anything out of the ordinary that may have occurred during the intraoperative period.

7.2.1. Critical care hand-off

As expected, patients transported to the ICU from the OR are often critically ill. Many institutions include a formal hand-off tool (paper-based or computerized) that must be completed prior to ICU transport. Utilization of these hand-off tools can serve not only as a checklist but also as an important means of communication that has been shown to improve patient safety and outcomes. The Accreditation Council for Graduate Medical Education has made hand-off communication education a requirement for all accredited teaching programs in the United States. The PACU is traditionally divided into phase I and phase II. The majority of patients who have received general or neuraxial anesthesia will transition from the OR to phase I PACU.

7.2.2. Phase I PACU

Phase I denotes readily available staff and equipment should the patient require life-saving interventions. This includes airway rescue and cardiopulmonary support. Patients will be monitored continuously in this setting with 1:1 nursing ratio for at least the first 15 minutes postoperatively.

7.2.3. Phase II PACU

Phase II PACU is a transition between intense monitoring to either home discharge or the hospital ward. Certain patients may be appropriate to bypass phase I PACU and fast-track to phase II PACU in order to reduce hospital time and facilitate early discharge. Candidates suitable for fast-track transition are those who have received monitored anesthesia care or peripheral regional anesthesia for their procedure; are awake, alert, and responsive; have stable vital signs; and are able to ambulate with minimal assistance. Their pain should be under control and they should not complain of any nausea. Ultimately, patient comorbidities, type of procedure, and clinical judgement determine whether a patient is appropriate for fast-tracking to phase II.

7.3. PACU discharge

Criteria are in place to guide the decision to transition a patient from phase I to phase II PACU. Aldrete criteria (Table 7.1) were established in 1970 to guide the initial decision to move a patient through phase I recovery. Patients require a score of 9 out of 10 to progress to the next phase of recovery. Several revisions of the scoring system such as the Post-anesthesia Discharge Scoring System (Table 7.2) have emerged based on advances in monitoring

Table 7.1. The Aldrete Score	
Activity	2 = moves 4 extremities voluntarily or on command 1 = moves 2 extremities voluntarily or on command 0 = unable to move extremities
Respiration	2 = breathes deeply and coughs freely 1 = dyspnea or limited breathing 0 = apneic
Circulation	2 = BP ± 20% of preanesthetic level 1 = BP ± 20–49% of preanesthetic level 0 = BP ± 50% of preanesthetic level
O$_2$ Saturation	2 = maintains O$_2$ saturation > 92% on room air 1 = needs supplemental O$_2$ to maintain saturation > 90% 0 = O$_2$ saturation < 90% even with supplemental O$_2$
Consciousness	2 = fully awake 1 = arousable on calling 0 = not responsive

Aldrete JA, Kroulik D. A postanesthetic recovery score. *Anesth Analg.* 1970;49:924–934.

Table 7.2. Modified Postanesthetic Discharge Scoring System

Vital Signs	2 = within 20% of preoperative value 1 = 20–40% of preoperative value 0 = 40% or more of preoperative value
Ambulation	2 = steady gait/no dizziness 1 = with assistance 0 = no ambulation/has dizziness
Nausea & vomiting	2 = minimal 1 = moderate, requiring treatment 0 = severe, requiring treatment
Pain	2 = minimal 1 = moderate, requiring treatment 0 = severe, requiring treatment
Surgical Bleeding	2 = minimal 1 = moderate 0 = severe

Chung F, Chan VW, Ong D. A postanesthetic discharge scoring system for home readiness after ambulatory surgery. *J Clin Anesth*. 1995;7:500–506.

technology and a growing number of ambulatory patients who discharge home. Nevertheless, all scoring systems focus on similar categories which include activity, respiration, circulation, color or oxygen saturation, and consciousness. These variables are assessed at 5, 15, 30, 45, and 60 minutes by the PACU nurse and finally at discharge by an anesthesia provider.

7.4. Postanesthesia evaluation

7.4.1. In PACU

While overseeing the PACU, residents will be asked to assess patients after anesthesia (Table 7.3). Remembering the "ABCs"—airway, breathing, and circulation—is a good way to start an assessment. After anesthesia, patients may have airway compromise including upper airway obstruction from residual sedation, stridor, or wheezing. Airway patency may need to be supported with jaw thrust, an oral airway, noninvasive positive pressure ventilation, or even reintubation. Respiratory drive may be diminished due to a combination of persistent inhaled anesthetics, opioids, or hypercarbia. Respiratory weakness may be seen from residual neuromuscular blockade and may require treatment with reversal agents such as sugammadex or neostigmine.

Hemodynamic instability may be present due to the nature of the surgery, blood loss, residual anesthetic, pain medications, or cardiac dysrhythmias. Patients may require fluid resuscitation,

Table 7.3. Common postanesthesia care unit complications	
o Hypertension	o Hypoxemia
o Pain	o Airway obstruction
o Anxiety	o Hypoventilation (narcotics,
o Poor control of blood pressure	sedatives, residual anesthesia)
at baseline	o Persistent neuromuscular
	blockade
Hypotension	o Atelectasis (obesity, low tidal
o Hypovolemia (bleeding,	volumes during surgery)
inadequate fluid	o Bronchospasm, COPD
administration, etc.)	exacerbation
o Vasodilation (drugs, rewarming)	o Pulmonary edema
o Ventricular dysfunction	o Pneumothorax
(perioperative MI, arrhythmia)	
o Sepsis	
o Pneumothorax (central line	
related, laparoscopy, etc.)	

COPD = chronic obstructive pulmonary disease; MI = myocardial infarction.

inotropic support, vasopressor or antiarrhythmic administration, blood transfusion, or even a return to the OR.

7.4.2. On nursing unit

Similar issues may carry over onto the nursing unit if they develop later in the postoperative course or are not adequately addressed in the PACU. Nurses may page the anesthesia resident about these issues.

7.4.3. By phone

During a phone assessment, it is important to triage calls and deal with the most life-threatening issues immediately. Airway and resuscitation equipment should be readily available in all areas of the hospital.

7.4.4. Considerations of care

Less immediately life-threatening PACU problems commonly include pain, nausea, hypothermia, and shivering. Multimodal approaches to pain are often more successful than single agents. These may include additional analgesic administration or acute pain service intervention with neuraxial or regional analgesic techniques. In coordination with the respective surgical service, a patient-controlled analgesia device may also be utilized for postoperative pain control. Postoperative nausea and vomiting (PONV) is a unique problem in the PACU, with patients often reporting PONV to be worse than postoperative pain. It can significantly prolong PACU or hospital stay and even lead to unanticipated hospital admission. The presence of risk factors (Box 7.2) can help identify those who may need prophylactic measures such as placement of a scopolamine patch. Similar to pain management,

Box 7.2 Important risk factors for postoperative nausea and vomiting

- Age: < 50 years
- Surgery: cholecystectomy, gynecologic surgery, laparoscopy, eye/inner ear surgery
- Gender: female
- History: previous postoperative nausea and vomiting, motion sickness, nonsmoker
- Intraoperative factors: use of volatile agents, duration of anesthesia
- Postoperative factors: use of opioids

Gan TJ, Diemunsch P, Habib AS, et al. Consensus guidelines for the management of postoperative nausea and vomiting. *Anesth Analg.* 2014;118(1):85–113.

a multifaceted approach to nausea is often more successful than single-agent administration. Examples of this include intravenous medications such as serotonin 5HT-3 receptor antagonists (ondansetron), steroids (dexamethasone), butyrophenones (haloperidol), NK-1 antagonists (aprepitant), antihistamines (promethazine), dopamine receptor antagonists (metoclopramide), or intramuscular ephedrine. Typical IV doses for average sized adults are 4 mg of ondansetron, 4 to 8 mg of dexamethasone, 10 mg of metoclopramide, 12.5 to 25 mg of promethazine, and 1 mg of haloperidol. Ensuring adequate hydration will also minimize postoperative nausea. Postoperative shivering can usually be treated with warm blankets, forced air warming, or IV meperidine administration.

7.5. Postanesthesia patient instructions for ambulatory patients

After meeting appropriate ambulatory surgery center discharge criteria (Table 7.3), the patient must have a responsible individual to accompany him or her home. This should be mandatory across accredited institutions in the United States and has been shown to reduce adverse outcomes and increase patient comfort and satisfaction. While the requirement to drink and void prior to discharge is no longer mandatory for most patients, written instructions and precautions must be provided to the patient, and he or she should have a responsible escort who can contact the hospital should a problem arise once the patient is discharged. Examples of potential problems include refractory pain, nausea, inability to tolerate fluids, or inability to urinate. In addition, patients should be warned of the dangers of driving, operating heavy machinery, or making important decisions within 24 hours after anesthesia and/or while continuing to take narcotic pain medications. Whenever regional anesthesia is performed, the patient should be given precautions to protect the limb with sensory block, begin analgesic medications before experiencing severe pain, and contact a provider in case of unresolved neurologic deficit.

With increasing life expectancy, the average age of the surgical population is rising. An elderly patient needs additional precautions upon PACU discharge. For instance, caregivers should be advised that because elderly patients are more sensitive to the respiratory depressant effect of opioids, which can manifest once they leave the PACU, extra vigilance is required. Caregivers should also be advised of postoperative cognitive decline, which can manifest as delirium, confusion, disorientation, and memory loss among other symptoms. The elderly are also at increased risk of hypothermia, falls, medication errors, and positioning injuries, which necessitate ensuring an adequate support system upon discharge as well as education of the caregivers to return to the hospital if these issues arise.

Another surgical population that requires additional instructions upon discharge from the PACU are patients with obstructive sleep apnea (OSA). Patients with OSA are prone to upper airway collapse leading to obstruction, especially after receiving opioids for postoperative pain. If they are already on a continuous positive airway pressure machine at home, they should be advised to continue the same therapy to prevent desaturation events. Efforts should be made to pursue opioid-sparing techniques such as the use of nonsteroidal anti-inflammatory drugs, acetaminophen, or regional anesthesia when appropriate for postoperative pain control in this population.

Further Reading

Aldrete JA, Kroulik D. A postanesthetic recovery score. *Anesth Analg.* 1970;49:924–934.

Chung F, Chan VW, Ong D. A postanesthetic discharge scoring system for home readiness after ambulatory surgery. *J Clin Anesth.* 1995;7:500–506.

Gan TJ, Diemunsch P, Habib AS, et al. Consensus guidelines for the management of postoperative nausea and vomiting. *Anesth Analg.* 2014;118(1):85–113.

Nicholau D. The postanesthesia care unit. In: Miller RD, ed. *Miller's Anesthesia,* 7th ed. Philadelphia: Churchill Livingstone; 2010:2707–2728.

Practice guidelines for postanesthetic care—An updated report by the American Society of Anesthesiologists Task Force on Postanesthetic Care. *Anesthesiology.* 2013;118:1–17.

Chapter 8

Specialty Practice Situations

Efrain Riveros-Perez and Mauricio Perilla

8.1. Anesthesia in remote locations

8.1.1. Anesthesia for gastrointestinal endoscopic procedures

Diagnosis and treatment techniques for gastrointestinal disorders have evolved over the last decade. As technology advances, so does the complexity of endoscopic procedures of the upper and lower gastrointestinal tract. The procedures have become more invasive, necessitating the participation of an interdisciplinary team of proceduralists, anesthesiologists, and nursing staff to ensure safe and high-quality patient care.

As the number and complexity of endoscopic gastrointestinal procedures continue to grow in the United States, the services of an anesthesiologist are often requested to facilitate the interventions, while also ensuring patient safety and comfort in an older and sicker population. The anesthetic techniques employed encompass a wide variety of possibilities ranging from minimal sedation to conscious sedation and general anesthesia (Box 8.1 Box 8.2).

Although most of the endoscopic interventions can be performed under sedation, some special circumstances such as a full stomach, depressed airway reflexes, a patient's inability to protect his or her airway, prone positioning, and long procedures with increased risk of aspiration of gastric contents warrant the use of general anesthesia.

Regardless of the chosen anesthetic technique, each patient should have a preoperative evaluation including a complete history and physical examination focusing on comorbidities, preoperative fasting, as well as risk factors for aspiration of gastric contents and full assessment of the airway, recognizing that tracheal intubation will always be a backup plan. When deep sedation is indicated, the anesthetic goals include ensuring patient comfort and analgesia, avoidance of patient movement during the procedure, preservation

Box 8.1 Characteristics of anesthetic procedures done in the endoscopy suite

- Remote location out of the traditional operating room setting
- Nursing staff trained in care of short endoscopic procedures, not necessarily in post-anesthesia care
- High case turnover
- Ambulatory patient population in a majority of cases
- Combination of low- and high-complexity procedures requiring customized anesthetic care
- American Society of Anesthesiologists physical status ranging from I to V that requires tailoring of anesthetic approaches

of spontaneous ventilation, and maintaining airway patency. Continuous assessment of respiratory pattern and capnographic waveform guide the anesthesiologist to titrate the anesthetic and to implement maneuvers to open the airway. These endpoints are usually achieved with the combination of a propofol infusion and titrated boluses of opioids such as fentanyl. Remifentanil infusions can also be administered; however, the anesthesia provider must be aware of the risk of apnea. Postprocedural analgesia is part of the anesthetic plan. Most endoscopic procedures are not particularly painful; however, some of these patients suffer from chronic pain conditions and provision of analgesia may be challenging.

When there is risk of aspiration, rapid sequence induction is indicated. Drainage of stomach contents after removing the endoscope

Box 8.2 Common endoscopic procedures requiring anesthesia management

Basic procedures:
- Esophagogastroduodenoscopy
- Colonoscopy
- Flexible sigmoidoscopy

Complex procedures:
- Endoscopic retrograde cholangiopancreatography
- Sphincterotomy, bile stone duct removal, biliary stents
- Esophageal varices banding
- Endoscopic ultrasound
- Esophageal stent/dilation
- Double balloon enteroscopy

is recommended before extubation. Prevention of postoperative nausea and vomiting (PONV) must be provided according to preoperative risk assessment. Discharge from the postanesthesia care unit must abide by institutional protocols and guidelines (Box 8.3).

8.1.2. Anesthesia for eye surgery

The main objectives of anesthetic care for ophthalmologic surgery are facilitation of the operation, patient comfort, rapid recovery, and mitigation of risks associated with the patient's condition. Most ophthalmologic procedures in the United States are performed under monitored anesthesia care (MAC), although in some instances, depending on unique patient characteristics or type of surgery, general anesthesia is indicated. When a MAC technique is employed, local or regional anesthesia must be provided to create favorable conditions to perform the operation. Some superficial procedures can be done with topical anesthesia, whereas interventions of deeper structures might require the use of retrobulbar, peribulbar, or sub-Tenon block.

The patient undergoing eye surgery presents several special challenges to the anesthesiologist. In addition to providing patient comfort and immobility, awareness of factors such as systemic effects of ocular medications, prevention and management of oculocardiac reflex, control of intraocular gas expansion, and smooth emergence are critical (Table 8.1).

Box 8.3 Anesthesia in the endoscopy suite: facts to remember	
Preanesthesia evaluation	History and physical examination Airway assessment Evaluation of aspiration risk Assessment of PONV risk Anesthetic plan Informed consent
Intraprocedure course	Monitored anesthesia care Airway patency Capnographic evidence of breathing General anesthesia Rapid sequence induction Hemodynamic stability Adequate anesthetic depth level Awake extubation
Postanesthesia care	Adequate analgesia PONV treatment Disposition

Table 8.1. Monitored anesthesia care and general anesthesia for eye surgery

MAC	General anesthesia
Minimal effect on intraocular pressure	Effect on intraocular pressure
Efficient use of OR	Longer time to recovery and discharge
Rapid recovery and discharge	Protection of the airway
Limited to short procedures	Higher risk of PONV
Risk of eye injury (ocular blocks)	Can be used if patient cannot remain still

PONV = postoperative nausea and vomiting.

8.1.2.1. Monitored anesthesia care

MAC techniques can be divided into two stages. The first stage consists of the provision of analgesia, amnesia, and hypnosis for a short period to facilitate the performance of ocular blocks. Depending on the institution, this stage might take place in the preoperative holding area. During this stage, airway equipment must be ready and checked, supplemental oxygen must be administered, and a patient's intravenous (IV) line must be in place. Propofol is the most commonly used medication at a dose between 0.5 and 0.75 mg/kg. At this dose range, apnea rarely occurs; however, equipment to assist ventilation should be by the bedside. The second stage corresponds to the maintenance phase. The patient has to be able to follow verbal commands and communicate with the surgical team. The anesthesiologist must reassure the patient and assess his or her ability to co-operate with the procedure by maintaining immobility. Small titrated doses of midazolam and a short-acting opioid can be used during this stage. Finally, since drapes are covering the patient's face, checking for closed pockets that put the patient at risk of fire formation or rebreathing is part of intraoperative management.

8.1.2.2. General anesthesia

The choice of induction agent for general anesthesia depends on the patient's characteristics, eye pathology, and planned procedure. Avoiding increases in ocular pressure is one of the main goals in ophthalmologic anesthesia. Stabilization of intraocular pressure requires judicious administration of opioids and IV lidocaine to mitigate the sympathetic response to laryngoscopy and intubation as well as muscle relaxants to eliminate the cough reflex. Securing the airway with a laryngeal mask airway in the absence of

> **Box 8.4 Intraoperative oculocardiac reflex management**
>
> Communicate with the surgeon
>
> Stop surgical stimulation
>
> Administer local lidocaine injection near extraocular muscles
>
> Administer atropine (0.01 mg/kg)
>
> Check depth of general anesthesia. Maintain normocapnia.

contraindications might be indicated; however, since access to the airway is restricted in eye surgery, the anesthesia provider must pay continuous attention to signs of laryngospasm and airway obstruction in these cases. The use of succinylcholine in ophthalmologic surgery is controversial. Succinylcholine is known to increase intraocular pressure and is contraindicated in most instances of ophthalmologic surgery; however, in full-stomach situations, the benefit of shortening the time of unprotected airway before tracheal intubation far outweighs the transient increase in ocular pressure. On the other hand, using rocuronium at four times the effective dose causes intubating conditions with an onset time similar to that of succinylcholine, making it a sound alternative in those challenging situations. If the procedure is shorter than the duration of action of rocuronium or if the patient becomes difficult to ventilate/intubate, muscle relaxation can be reversed with sugammadex.

Nitrous oxide has limited use in eye surgery due to increased risk of PONV and should be avoided in vitreoretinal detachment procedures where bubbles of sulfur hexachloride are created. Finally, eye surgery requires the anesthesiologist to be positioned away from the head, warranting extra caution with circuit disconnections, airway obstruction, and accidental extubation risks. Oculocardiac reflex, which is defined clinically as a decrease in heart rate following pressure to the globe or traction of the ocular muscles, is relatively common during ophthalmologic surgery. Treatment of this phenomenon is described in Box 8.4.

8.1.3. Anesthesia in the electrophysiology lab

In the past, electrophysiology (EP) procedures were performed for diagnostic purposes only. More recently, interventions in the EP lab have evolved to include technologies that are more sophisticated and include a variety of therapeutic modalities. The fact that these procedures are performed in remote locations and that the patient population typically has significant cardiac and noncardiac morbidities makes anesthesia in the EP lab very challenging.

Box 8.5 Commonly encountered arrhythmias in the EP lab

Paroxysmal supraventricular tachycardia

Atrioventricular nodal reentrant tachycardia

Atrioventricular reciprocating tachycardia—Wolf-Parkinson-White arrhythmia

Atrial tachycardia

Atrial flutter

Atrial fibrillation

Premature ventricular contractions/ventricular tachycardia

Commonly encountered arrhythmias in the EP lab are listed in Box 8.5. In addition to the mapping and treatment of arrhythmias, other types of procedures such as implantation of pacemakers and defibrillator devices take place in the EP lab.

Indications for implantation of pacemakers and defibrillator devices are expanding with the advent of newer technologies and the increased number of patients with cardiac morbidities associated with rhythm disturbances. See Box 8.6 for the preprocedure checklist for automated implantable cardiac devices.

Anesthetic considerations for EP procedures are multiple and are summarized in Box 8.7.

The choice of anesthetic technique for EP procedures is based on several factors including patient characteristics and preferences, the need for complete immobility, and duration of the intervention.

Box 8.6 Preprocedure checklist for automated implantable cardiac devices

Complete set up of the procedure room for possible general anesthesia

Consider an arterial line for continuous monitoring

Have adequate large-bore vascular access

Type and cross two units of packed red blood cells

Attach and check temporary cardiac pacing

Review last dose of anticoagulation therapy and coagulation status

Equipment and personnel for immediate sternotomy readily available

Administer antibiotics

Sterile preparation and draping for median sternotomy and femoral access

Box 8.7 What an anesthesiologist in the EP lab must remember
Non-tipping tables (may consider induction on transport bed)
High density of equipment and cables/electrodes in the room
Transesophageal echocardiography may be required in some procedures (general anesthesia)
Routine use of vasopressors to sustain blood pressure
Heparin administered after transseptal puncture (maintain activated clotting time between 250 and 300 s)
Patient immobility is critical in some cases (monitor muscle relaxation, decreased chest excursion)
Nasogastric tube may be needed to highlight esophageal anatomy during procedure
Esophageal temperature monitor to warn about risk of esophageal injury
Close monitoring of fluid balance
Smooth extubation to prevent groin hematoma

When sedation is chosen, a minimal to moderate approach is recommended to facilitate mapping. Dexmedetomidine and propofol infusions have been successfully used in most procedures; however, propofol may slow atrioventricular nodal conduction. General anesthesia with volatile anesthetics is equivalent to total IV techniques with the exception of cases with atrioventricular nodal re-entry tachycardia in which halogenated agents suppress arrhythmic activity. There is evidence in favor of utilizing general anesthesia for atrial fibrillation ablation. General anesthesia reduces the prevalence of pulmonary vein reconnection. This finding could be attributed to better patient immobility and more accurate mapping and catheter stability. Postanesthesia considerations are listed in Box 8.8.

Box 8.8 Relevant postanesthesia aspects after EP procedures
Nursing staff needs adequate training
Be vigilant of signs of cardiac tamponade (if necessary perform transthoracic echocardiogram)
Pain control with oral medications (avoid NSAIDs due to risk of bleeding)
Evaluate dyspnea (atrial stunning versus fluid overload or myocardial ischemia)

8.1.4. Anesthesia in the cardiac catheterization lab

Cardiac catheterization procedures have increased exponentially. The involvement of the anesthesiologist in these procedures is becoming an integral part of perioperative management in certain high-risk patient populations. The catheterization lab is a remote location and represents a foreign environment to the anesthesiologist. The room is normally crowded with different kinds of equipment, and the work area for the anesthesiologist is usually limited. Becoming familiar with the environment and maintaining constant communication with the cardiologist, technicians, and nursing staff is essential during the different stages of the procedure.

The anesthesiologist must be aware of the location of all anesthesia equipment, emergency supplies, and medications as well as established lines to call for help should the need arise. The same standards for providing safe anesthesia that apply in regular operating rooms (ORs) should also be applied in the catheterization lab. The patient is a distance from the anesthesia provider during the intervention. Therefore, extra-long line tubing and gas circuits are needed to avoid accidental pulling of lines and tubes and tangling with pieces of equipment. At the same time, an organized arrangement of lines and tubes permits easy access to ports and to the airway. Regarding monitors, all these procedures must comply with the American Society of Anesthesiologists standards.

General anesthesia and MAC can be administered in the catheterization lab. The choice of the anesthetic technique depends on the type and duration of the procedure. It is recommended that a discussion with the cardiologist regarding the anesthetic needs for the procedure take place before the patient is rolled to the room. General anesthesia is indicated for long procedures especially when the need for cessation of ventilation is anticipated. Although in many instances patients undergo these procedures with sedation, most adult patients receive it from trained nursing staff. The anesthesiologist intervenes only in pediatric cases and in cases of adult patients in severely compromised medical conditions. Common procedures performed in the cardiac catheterization lab are listed in Box 8.9.

Exposure to radiation during fluoroscopy is significant in the cardiac catheterization suite. The side effects of repeated exposure to significant doses of radiation range from skin irritation to cellular mutation, cancer, and teratogenicity. The anesthesiologist must wear a radiation dosimeter during the radiation phase of the intervention. Exposure to radiation must be limited by application of three principles: keeping the maximum possible distance from the source, minimizing time of exposure, and shielding by using lead aprons and collars. Acrylic stands are recommended to further

Box 8.9 Procedures commonly performed in the catheterization lab
Percutaneous intervention
Percutaneous closure of septal defects
Transcatheter cardiac valve stents
Electrophysiological studies
Implantable cardioverter/defibrillator

limit exposure of the anesthesia personnel. It is also advisable to limit the administration of bolus anesthetic medications and rely more on infusions and inhaled agents.

Contrast agents are routinely used in the catheterization lab and can cause allergic reactions/anaphylaxis and nephrotoxicity. The contrast solutions can be classified as ionic and non-ionic. Non-ionic agents are associated with a lower incidence of vasodilation and electrocardiographic changes. Adequate preprocedural hydration is of paramount importance to mitigate the risk of renal injury. Also important in this regard is limiting the total dose of contrast. N-acetylcysteine is not recommended for preventing or treating contrast-induced nephropathy.

8.1.5. Anesthesia in the radiology suite

With the advancement of imaging technologies and the development of radiology-aided interventional procedures, the number of procedures requiring anesthesia care in radiology suites has steadily increased over the last decade. Neurointerventional and body interventional radiology, in addition to magnetic resonance imaging (MRI) and tomography, are examples of settings in which anesthesiologists are required to participate. As is the case with other out-of-the-operating-room contexts, radiology suites are located in remote areas of the hospital, and providing anesthesia in these unfamiliar settings presents unique challenges (Box 8.10).

MRI diagnostic studies employ a magnetic field that affects the polarity of water molecules in a differential manner between tissues and fluids, producing an image that can be reconstructed. The patient must be interrogated about MRI-incompatible implants or devices before proceeding to perform the study. Confinement of the patient in a tight space and a high level of noise are factors that warrant anesthetic interventions in selected patients. The anesthesia provider must be cleared for MRI compatibility following safety protocols. Implantable electronic devices such as pacemakers and implantable defibrillators are generally contraindicated in the MRI suite.

Box 8.10 Factors influencing anesthetic care in the radiology suite

Patient-related factors:
- Mental status (anxiety, claustrophobia, confusion)
- Ability to be in supine position for prolonged time (cardiopulmonary disease, pain)

Procedure-related factors:
- Complexity and duration of the study/intervention
- Distance between anesthesiologist and patient (airway, IV access)
- Need for immobility and periods of apnea
- MRI compatibility and radiation exposure
- Contrast utilization

The choice of anesthesia technique depends on the patient characteristics and type of procedure. Utilization of MRI-compatible monitors is mandatory as is placement of the anesthesia machine at a safe distance from the magnet with long gas circuits. Ideally, the patient should be induced in a separate room and then transferred to the MRI suite on an MRI-compatible gurney. If an IV anesthetic technique is considered, an MRI-compatible infusion pump with remote controls is recommended. Extreme attention to patient positioning is necessary, and it is important to avoid pressure point injuries. A trial with extreme position of the table is recommended to ensure sufficient line and circuit length.

Neurointerventional radiology is a fast-growing field in which anesthesiologists usually participate. Patients requiring these types of procedures present unique challenges (Box 8.11). Patient neurological status may change rapidly, and multiple comorbidities impact the anesthetic plan. During the study, an initial set of fluoroscopic images with IV contrast is obtained to serve as a reference frame (mask) on which subsequent images are superimposed. For the technique to be successful, patient immobility is critical. If the patient is under sedation, he or she must be able to follow commands and hold still during critical moments of the procedure. If the patient is unable to comply, general anesthesia is a better alternative.

Interventional radiology procedures are used for both diagnostic and therapeutic purposes. Many patients undergo sedation for these procedures, and intervention of the anesthesiologist is required for high-risk, complex cases (Box 8.12).

Intracranial aneurysm rupture

Arterial dissection

Retroperitoneal hemorrhage

Coil migration/fracture

Cerebral vasospasm

Contrast reaction

Hemodynamic instability

Airway compromise

8.2. Emergency airway out of the OR: Role of the anesthesiologist

Urgent and emergent airway management is often required outside of the OR. Inadequate management of the airway in settings where tracheal intubation is not routine can lead to significant adverse events. A well-established institutional pathway addressing team activation has been associated with better outcomes in airway emergencies. The team should consist of a leader (anesthesia provider or intensivist) and a respiratory therapist. Airway equipment should be available in all hospital locations, and every anesthesia department should have an "emergency airway box"

Box 8.12 High-risk interventional radiology cases requiring anesthesia

Aortic endoleak repair

Embolization of bleeding gastrointestinal vessels

Embolization of uterine/hypogastric arteries in obstetric hemorrhage

Pulmonary artery occlusion in life-threatening hemoptysis

Trauma-associated bleeding

Complex vascular stenting procedures

Occlusion of arteriovenous malformations

Drainage procedures for urosepsis and biliary sepsis

Drainage of pleural and abdominal collections in severely ill patients with basic and emergency airway devices as well as induction and emergency medications. A process for maintenance and inventory of the box according to institutional guidelines must be in place.

Patients requiring tracheal intubation out of the OR are usually critically ill and have poor cardiopulmonary reserve. Additionally, the physical location is generally not set up to perform this type of procedure. The anesthesia provider must be aware of all the equipment necessary in the room including oxygen source and suction. Of special importance is the identification of personnel including nurses and staff who are available to bring additional equipment or to activate alarm systems.

The initial approach to the patient must focus on airway patency and optimizing oxygenation. Given the poor pulmonary reserve, it is advisable to use a bag valve mask with supplemental oxygen and, if necessary, gently assist ventilation, keeping in mind the risk of aspiration of gastric contents. At this point, a brief history gathering is important, focusing on critical aspects such as the cause of respiratory deterioration, baseline condition, acuity of the situation, allergies, and history of difficult airway. It is important to assess the feasibility of alternatives to intubation such as noninvasive positive pressure ventilation based on the patient's conditions and absence of contraindications. If the patient requires tracheal intubation, a quick airway assessment is necessary to determine the course of action in terms of airway access technique and the feasibility of intubation in the awake patient versus after induction of anesthesia. Before instrumenting the airway, ensure that the items listed in (Box 8.13) are evaluated. Box 8.14 lists the recommended equipment required in an airway cart or box used for securing the airway outside the OR.

If the patient is to be intubated awake, the airway should be adequately topicalized. The availability of a fiberoptic bronchoscope

Box 8.13 Checklist

- Location of additional oxygen sources
- Availability of airway devices (to follow difficult airway algorithms)
- Availability of working suction
- Availability of support personnel
- Availability of line to call for help
- Ready availability of surgeon for potential surgical airway
- Availability of emergency medications and induction agents
- Disposition after intubation (intensive care unit)

Box 8.14 Recommended airway cart/box equipment
Direct laryngoscope with different blade types and sizes
Videolaryngoscope
Supraglottic devices
Flexible fiberoptic bronchoscope
Endotracheal tubes of different sizes
End-tidal carbon dioxide detector (colorimetric)
Surgical airway tray
Airway adjuncts (elastic bougie, tube exchangers)

and videolaryngoscope should be verified. If general anesthesia is chosen, rapid sequence induction is indicated, provided that there are no contraindications. Hemodynamic stability must be monitored throughout the process and maintained with IV fluids and vasoactive medications. Verification of expired carbon dioxide is standard of care and can be obtained with capnographic monitors or colorimetric methods. Once the patient is intubated, communication with the primary team and the intensive care team is recommended, and a detailed evaluation of the overall organ system condition should take place. Coordination of transfer of care must include the nursing staff and the teams involved.

Further Reading

Anderson R, Harukuni I, Sera V. Anesthetic considerations for electrophysiologic procedures. *Anesthesiol Clin*. 2013;31:479–489.

Apfelbaum JL, Caplan RA, Barker SJ, et al. Practice advisory for the prevention and management of operating room fires: an updated report by the American Society of Anesthesiologists Task Force on Operating Room Fires. *Anesthesiology*.2013; 118:271–290.

Chambers CE1, Fetterly KA, Holzer R, Lin PJ, Blankenship JC, Balter S, Laskey WK. Radiation safety program for the cardiac catheterization laboratory. *Catheter Cardiovasc Interv*. 2011;77:546–556.

Di Biase L, Conti S, Mohanty P, et al. General anesthesia reduces the prevalence of pulmonary vein reconnection during repeat ablation when compared with conscious sedation: results from a randomized study. *Heart Rhythm*. 2011;8:368–372.

Eke T, Thompson JR. The National Survey of Local Anaesthesia for Ocular Surgery. II. Safety profiles of local anaesthesia techniques. *Eye*. 1999;13(Pt. 2):196–204.

Fanning GL. Orbital regional anesthesia. *Ophthalmol Clin North Am*. 2006;19:221–232.

Joung KW, Yang KH, Shin WJ, Song MH, Ham K, Jung SC, Lee DH, Suh DC. Anesthetic consideration for neurointerventional procedures. *Neurointervention.* 2014;9:72–77.

Metzner J, Posner KL, Domino KB. The risk and safety of anesthesia at remote locations: the US closed claims analysis. *Curr Opin Anaesthesiol.* 2009;22(4):502–508.

Shook DC, Gross W. Offsite anesthesiology in the cardiac catheterization lab. *Curr Opin Anaesthesiol.* 2007;20:352–358.

Tetzlaff JE, Vargo JJ, Maurer W. Nonoperating room anesthesia for the gastrointestinal endoscopy suite. *Anesthesiol Clin.* 2014;32:387–394.

The 2007 Recommendations of the International Commission on Radiological Protection. ICRP publication 103. *Ann ICRP.* 2007;37:1–332.

Veenith T, Coles JP. Anaesthesia for magnetic resonance imaging and positron emission tomography. *Curr Opin Anaesthesiol.* 2011;24:451–458.

Chapter 9

Continuous Quality Improvement

Sarah M. I. Cartwright

9.1. Terminology

Continuous quality improvement (CQI) is a concept that crosses multiple industries and has gained momentum in health care. The Institute of Medicine (IOM) charged provider groups, including anesthesiologists, to change the delivery of health care through the triple aim of improving patient experience, reducing costs, and improving clinical outcomes. To achieve this measure, the provider must become skilled in continuously improving each opportunity over the previous one. Recently, understanding that the concepts of CQI can be received as burdensome to the provider, the IOM has changed the triple aim to the quadruple aim of improving patient outcomes, while decreasing costs, and improving patient and provider experience in the process.

9.1.1. Quality in health care

Introduction to the concepts of quality vary between provider groups, but, seemingly, all provider groups agree that evidence-based approaches to care improve outcomes. This improvement cycle dynamics began with the recognition of concepts of quality in terms of objectively measuring incidents and reviewing them against established practice benchmarks. The IOM defined health care quality as "the degree to which health care services for individuals and populations increase the likelihood of desired health outcomes and are consistent with current professional knowledge." Perioperative surgical patients provide a unique population that requires expert care by anesthesia providers, care that is delivered through evidence-based practice. This constitutes quality anesthesia health care.

The American Society of Anesthesiologists (ASA) defines the expectation of anesthesiology practice through the publication of practice standards, guidelines, advisories, and statements, designed with patient safety and advancement of professional practice in mind. These guidelines and consensus statements give the anesthesia provider a high degree of current professional knowledge related to the practice of anesthesiology, consistent with the charge of the IOM.

The Anesthesia Quality Institute (AQI) was established to assist providers and practice groups to achieve benchmarking both internal to their peers and external from practice to practice. AQI provides voice to ASA's aim to develop "pertinent, meaningful measures, ongoing analysis of evidence-based practice parameters, review and updating of older practice parameters, and retirement of parameters no longer applicable."

Quality as a measure is based on the understanding of the defined best practice and conversion into metrics that can be measured. These measures, referred to as benchmarks, indicate how often the expected outcome occurs per opportunity. For instance, the evidence supports smoking cessation as a contributor to improved outcomes of care in the perioperative population. A quality measure for this evidence-based practice could be expressed as frequency of smoking cessation counseling encounters for identified tobacco users older than 18 years of age. Mathematically the measure would be expressed as n smoking cessation encounters/n smokers identified.

9.1.2. Continuous quality improvement

CQI is a structured approach to problem-solving that encourages anesthesiologists to ask the following questions about their practice: "What did I do today? What went well? What can I do better?" This cyclic questioning is used to generate trends and focus improvement activities.

9.2. Structured methodology and tools

A strength inherent to CQI is the systematic approach to problem-solving. There are several methodologies to achieve continuous improvement, each with its own merits. Regardless of the methodology used, the structure behind the process is the same.

When considering the scientific method, the process begins with asking a question. Similarly, with CQI the process begins with a question of improvement. Following the inquiry process, background research is done to understand the current state of the problem, followed by the creation of a hypothesis to be tested with an experience. Then, depending on the result of the test, the results are reported and a new experiment is begun. This systematic approach to problem-solving is modeled on the concepts used in the development of the Toyota Production System, the

Deming/Shewart (PDSA/PDCA) systems thinking approach, lean, six sigma, lean-six sigma, and multiple others.

9.2.1. Lean

Lean as a term was coined in 1988 by John Krafcik in the article "Triumph of the Lean Production System." This methodology looks at systems processes and targets wastes or deficiencies within the process that utilized resources without providing a return (value) for the efforts. This concept has been embraced by industry and manufacturing and has moved into health care to assist in work standardization and cost reduction. A Google search with the terms "lean thinking in health care" produced 1.28 million unique results in November 2017. This concept is popularizing in response to high costs and limited reimbursements in health care. The Institute for Healthcare Improvement white paper on "Going Lean in Health Care," published in 2005, states that "whether building a car or providing health care for a patient, workers must rely on multiple, complex processes to accomplish their tasks and provide value to the customer or patient. Wastes of money, time, supplies, or good will decrease value." Wastes are "responsible for work delays and added costs" (Connolly, *Washington Post,* June 4, 2005).

9.2.2. Six sigma

While lean focuses on wastes within processes, six-sigma methodology helps with the reduction of variations between users of a system toward a single outcome. One example of application of this methodology in anesthesia is the implementation of the systematic use of a hand-off tool between providers to minimize variation between user groups (the information may be different, but the process of relaying the information would be the same). In comparison with six sigma, lean methodology is more intuitive and produces results that are quickly seen, whereas six sigma may require advanced tools and long-term studies to show improvements.

9.3. Quality improvement tools

9.3.1. Outcome measures

Outcome measures are discrete data points that can be described in units of measure. These specific measures deltas are useful to follow up on the gaps between the current state of the problem and desired outcomes. Definition of outcomes must take into consideration that the more specific the outcome is, the more complete the data set will be. "Better" is not measurable, "soon" is not a timescale, and "some" is not a number.

9.3.2. Project charter

A project charter is a document that assists individuals within a project team to understand the beginning and end of their efforts, and the rationale behind why they are working on the project.

It is important to use a concept document such as a project charter to help the team ensure that the correct individuals who can contribute to the process are part of the project.

Project charters typically consist of elements that may be specific to organizations.

• Project Title: Descriptor of the project.
• Problem Statement: What is the problem you are trying to solve?
• Goal Statement: How will you know you have solved the problem? What's your outcome?
• Scope In/Out: What is the beginning and endpoint of change? Is it something you can effect?
• Business Case and Benefits: What is happening now; what will happen if the change occurs? Is there a return on investment (better outcomes, less cost, etc.)?
• Timeline: How long will it take to do each part of the project?
• Resources/Budget: What will it take to complete the project? Resources include people, time, budget, technology, leadership agreement.
• Team Members/Stakeholders: Who is part of the change process? Who will be affected by the change process? Who has the power to say "no"?

Completing each step of the charter will help the group focus on the problem to be solved. It is easy to have the group become focused on issues outside of their control and/or purpose, which can decrease the functionality of the team. A charter is a snapshot document that creates agreement of purpose and scope of influence.

9.3.3. Voice of the customer translation matrix

When looking at process improvement tools and concepts that were designed for the manufacturing or business models, the terminology may seem out of place in the health care arena. The term "customer" is often observed within the tools, but the health care provider may substitute the population that is being observed for the term "customer." This could be a patient, a provider, a team, or a system.

In this tool, the voice of the customer assists the project team members in understanding the issues heard into actionable concepts or terminologies that assist in codification and planning (Table 9.1).

Table 9.1. Voice of the customer translation matrix		
Customer Comment (What was said?)	Gathering More Understanding (Why was that said?)	Customer Requirement (What is wanted?)
Example: I'm tired of waiting.	Example: Patient is waiting too long.	Example: Enter OR within 60 minutes of arrival to preop prep area.

This tool assists the project team to determine key take-away messages. This translation matrix takes "complaints" and turns them into "actions for resolution."

9.3.4. SIPOC matrix

Project teams must understand processes in terms of inputs and outputs to be able to follow workflows adequately. These workflows could be physical actions as people move through a process, concepts, information flows, or system functions. Each action has a reaction that affects the next action in line. Without understanding the flow of this information/action, any change could create additional concerns in processes before or after the area of influence.

A tool to assist the team in understanding these concepts is shown in Table 9.2. SIPOC is an acronym that stands for supplier, inputs, process, outputs, and customer. This table allows for a cross-venue understanding of basic flows with major processes and impactful subprocesses defined.

This SIPOC table maps out processes and identifies actions and stakeholders.

9.3.5. Data collection plan

All informed decisions begin with data. Data are then codified into information that is then actionable for change. This also helps ensure that the project team has an understanding of the aim/purpose of the project and what the measures are that prove success or failure (Agency for Healthcare Research and Quality, 2016).

A data collection plan is used to ensure that the most appropriate data are collected and that everyone agrees as to the type and purpose of the collection. By utilizing this tool, while creating measurements and metrics, the group develops a common language set for the project. It also allows for alignment between purpose, actions, and responsibilities. Baseline data are key to understand if a change occurred and to provide measurable outcomes.

Table 9.2. SIPOC matrix

S Supplier (Who brings the supplies to the area of need?)	I Inputs (What is needed for a process to begin? Could be people, actions, information.)	P Process (What are the steps in the process as you currently understand them?)	O Outputs (What is the outcome that occurs if the process is completed?)	C Customer (Who is the receiver of the outputs?)
Example: Patients Anesthesiologist Surgeon RNs	Example: A surgery order. Anesthesia supplies, medications, equipment, and technology. Room for patient. RNs to care for patient.	Example: Patient arrives for surgery. Patient taken to room to change clothes. RN completes assessment. Anesthesia completes/ documents assessment, exam, orders. RN completes orders. Patient ready for surgery.	Example: Patient taken to OR ready for anesthesia/surgery.	Surgical Patient. Surgeon. Anesthesiologist. OR team.

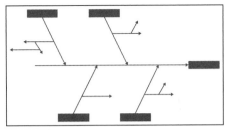

Figure 9.1. Fishbone diagram

9.3.6. Fishbone diagram

Fishbone diagrams, also known as Ishikawa and cause/effect diagrams, offer the project team a tool to organize data into major and minor themes. These diagrams work backward from a known outcome (effect) and assist in structuring potential causes (Figure 9.1).

Typical structures for the major themes can be remembered in various groupings, but any heading for a project is acceptable. The key is to ensure that the project group understands the categories and can explain the rationale behind choosing them.

Examples of category headers include the following.

Methods	Materials/Supplies	Machinery/Equipment	People/Staff
Policies	Procedures/Skills	Plant/Place of Work	Measurement/Metrics

Further Reading

Going lean in health care. IHI Innovation Series white paper. Cambridge, MA: Institute for Healthcare Improvement; 2005. Available at www.IHI.org.

Quality Improvement. Schaumburg, IL: American Society of Anesthesiologists; 2018. (Available at http://asahq.org/quality-and-practice-management/quality-and-regulatory-affairs).

Talking Quality. Rockville, MD: Agency for Healthcare Research and Quality; 2016. (Available at https://www.ahrq.gov/professionals/quality-patient-safety/talkingquality/index.html).

Glossary

Nadine Odo

This glossary defines terms commonly encountered during the first clinical anesthesia year.

ABCs—the acronym for Airway, Breathing, and Chest compressions (circulation).

Accreditation Council for Graduate Medical Education (ACGME)—the governing body responsible for accrediting the majority of graduate medical training programs for physicians in the United States.

Aldrete score—a commonly used scale for determining the safe discharge of patients from the postanesthesia care unit either to the postsurgical ward or to the second-stage (phase II) recovery area.

American Board of Anesthesiology (ABA)—one of the 24 medical specialty boards that constitutes the American Board of Medical Specialties; sets standards and examinations for the accreditation of board-certified anesthesiologists who are coming to the end of their residency and fellowship training.

Amnesia—loss of memory.

Analgesia—relief from or prevention of pain.

Anesthesia—a state of temporary induced loss of sensation or awareness. It may include analgesia, paralysis (muscle relaxation), amnesia, or unconsciousness.

Anesthesia breathing system—delivers oxygen and anesthetic gases to patients and eliminates carbon dioxide. It consists of a tubing to direct fresh gas flow, an adjustable pressure-limiting valve to control pressure within the system and allow scavenging of waste gas, and a reservoir bag to store gas and assist with ventilation.

Anesthesia care team (ACT)—consists of anesthesiologists, supervising qualified nonphysician anesthesia providers, and/or resident physicians who are training in the provision of anesthesia care.

Anesthesia delivery system—comprises the anesthesia machine, anesthesia vaporizer(s), ventilator, breathing circuit, and waste gas scavenging system.

Anesthesia information management systems (AIMS)—the hardware/software solution that interfaces with the intraoperative patient monitors, allowing the automatic and reliable collection, storage, and presentation of patient data during the perioperative period.

Anesthesia Knowledge Test—a series of examinations that are administered at different time intervals during residency training, designed to assess a resident's progress in knowledge.

Anxiolysis—the use of medication to decrease anxiety.

Arterial line—a thin catheter inserted into an artery to monitor blood pressure directly and in real time (rather than by intermittent and indirect measurement) and to obtain samples for arterial blood gas analysis.

BASIC examination—the first in the series of exams, offered to residents at the end of the first clinical anesthesia year. It focuses on the scientific basis of clinical anesthesia practice and concentrates on content areas such as pharmacology, physiology, anatomy, anesthesia equipment, and monitoring.

Bispectral index (BIS)—a depth of anesthesia monitor.

Bougie—an introducer with an angled tip designed to assist with endotracheal tube placement during difficult intubations.

Burnout—a state of chronic stress that leads to physical and emotional exhaustion, cynicism and detachment, feelings of ineffectiveness, and lack of accomplishment.

Cardiac catheterization—a procedure used to diagnose and treat cardiovascular conditions by inserting a long thin tube called a catheter into an artery or vein in the groin, neck, or arm and threaded through the blood vessels to the heart.

Electrophysiology study—a detailed evaluation of the electrical activity of the heart to find where an arrhythmia (abnormal heartbeat) is coming from.

Emergence—the transition from the anesthetized state to full consciousness.

Extubation—the removal of the endotracheal tube and disconnecting the patient from mechanical ventilation.

Fire triad—the three components required for a fire to occur: an oxidizer, an ignition source, and fuel.

Fluid resuscitation/management—replenishing bodily fluid lost through sweating, bleeding, fluid shifts, or other pathologic processes.

Functional residual capacity (FRC)—the volume of air present in the lungs at the end of passive expiration.

Goal-directed therapy—a technique involving intensive monitoring and aggressive management of perioperative hemodynamics in patients with a high risk of morbidity and mortality.

Hand-off—a transfer and acceptance of patient care responsibility achieved through effective communication.

Hemolytic transfusion reaction—a serious complication that can occur after a blood transfusion when the red blood cells given during the transfusion are destroyed by the person's immune system.

Hypnotic agents—a class of psychoactive drugs whose primary function is to induce sleep; commonly used in the treatment of insomnia (sleeplessness) or surgical anesthesia.

Induction—the administration of a drug or combination of drugs at the beginning of an anesthetic that results in a state of general anesthesia.

Informed consent—permission typically granted by a patient to a doctor for treatment with full knowledge of the possible risks and benefits.

Inspired oxygen fraction (FiO$_2$)—the fraction of inspired oxygen. For example, the fraction of inspired oxygen in air is 21%.

Interventional radiology—a range of techniques that relies on the use radiological image guidance (x-ray fluoroscopy, ultrasound, computed tomography, or magnetic resonance imaging) to precisely target therapy.

Intubation—the process of inserting an endotracheal tube through the mouth into the airway. This is done to place a patient on a ventilator to assist with breathing during anesthesia, sedation, or severe illness.

In-Training Examination—a computer-based exam with 200 multiple-choice questions that is administered each year to all physicians enrolled in anesthesiology residency training programs. Residency programs administer the four-hour exam at their sites.

Joint Commission—an independent, not-for-profit organization in collaboration with other stakeholders that accredits and certifies health care organizations and programs in the United States with the goal of improving quality of health care and maintaining standards.

Laryngoscope—a rigid endoscope equipped with a light source that is inserted in the mouth to facilitate intubation and examination of oropharynx and vocal cords.

Laryngospasm—sudden closure of the vocal cords causing cessation of ventilation, which may be precipitated by light anesthesia and secretions and can occur at the time of extubation.

Lithiotomy position—positioning of an individual's feet above or at the same level as the hips (often in stirrups), with the perineum positioned at the edge of an examination table.

Local anesthetic systemic toxicity (LAST)—central nervous system and cardiovascular system side effects from administration of local anesthetics.

Maintenance, anesthesia—phase of anesthesia between induction and emergence involving maintaining appropriate depth of anesthesia and monitoring for and treating intraoperative complications.

Maintenance of Certification in Anesthesiology (MOCA)—a web-based learning platform that provides physician anesthesia providers with opportunities to continuously learn and demonstrate proficiencies to provide better patient care.

Malignant hyperthermia—severe allergic reaction which can occur after exposure to anesthetic agents in susceptible patients, leading to fever, rigidity, rhabdomyolysis, and acidosis.

Mallampati score—used to predict the ease of endotracheal intubation.

Mean arterial pressure (MAP)—the average pressure in a patient's arteries during one cardiac cycle. It is considered a better indicator of perfusion to vital organs than systolic blood pressure.

Mechanical ventilation—mode of supporting ventilation using positive pressure, which can be invasive or noninvasive and is delivered via ventilator.

Mendelson's syndrome/pulmonary aspiration—a pneumonitis caused by aspiration of gastric contents during anesthesia, especially during pregnancy.

Minimal alveolar concentration (MAC)—the concentration of anesthetic gases in the lungs needed to prevent movement (motor response) in 50% of subjects in response to surgical stimulus (pain). MAC compares the strengths, or potency, of anesthetic gases.

Model for End-stage Liver Disease (MELD)—a predictor of disease severity and likely survival in patients awaiting liver transplant.

National Surgical Quality Improvement Program (NSQIP)—the leading nationally validated, risk-adjusted, outcomes-based program to measure and improve the quality of surgical care.

Peak inspiratory pressure—the highest level of pressure applied to the lungs during inhalation. In mechanical ventilation, the number reflects a positive pressure in centimeters of water pressure (cmH_2O).

Positive end-expiratory pressure—the pressure in the lungs (alveolar pressure) above atmospheric pressure (the pressure outside of the body) that exists at the end of expiration.

Postanesthesia care unit (PACU)—a care unit where patients who had received anesthesia are closely monitored (vital signs) and where their pain is managed and fluids given.

Postanesthetic Discharge Scoring System—a scale for determining when patients can be safely discharged from the postanesthesia care unit either to the postsurgical ward or to the second-stage (phase II) recovery area.

Postoperative cognitive decline (POCD)—a decline in cognitive function that may last from a few days to a few weeks and in rare cases may persist for several months after surgery.

Postoperative nausea and vomiting (PONV)—typically used to describe nausea and/or vomiting or retching in the postanesthesia care unit and in the immediate 24 postoperative hours.

Preanesthesia testing—helps prepare patients for surgery and ensures that facilities meet regulatory requirements for documentation.

Rapid sequence induction (RSI)—an established method of inducing anesthesia in patients who are at risk of aspiration of gastric contents into the lungs. The sequence involves the rapid administration of an induction agent whilst applying cricoid pressure, immediately followed by a fast-acting muscle relaxant with the aim to quickly achieve intubation conditions traditionally without the need for bag-mask ventilation.

Recruitment maneuver—a transient increase in transpulmonary pressure designed to open up collapsed airless alveoli.

Revised cardiac risk index (RCRI)—a tool used to estimate a patient's risk of perioperative cardiac complications.

Risk stratification—the process of categorizing patient populations into high-risk, moderate-risk, and low-risk tiers.

Scavenging system (anesthetic gas)—collects and removes waste gases from the patient's breathing circuit and the ventilation circuit.

Sedation—the administration of a sedative drug to produce a state of calm or sleep.

Surgical site infection (SSI)—an infection that occurs after surgery in the part of the body where the surgery took place.

Thyromental distance (TMD)—measured from the thyroid notch to the tip of the jaw with the head extended.

Time out—represents the final recapitulation and reassurance of accurate patient identity, surgical site, and planned procedure.

Transfusion-related acute lung injury (TRALI)—a serious blood transfusion complication characterized by the acute onset of noncardiogenic pulmonary edema following transfusion of blood products.

Vaporizer—a device generally attached to an anesthetic machine which delivers a given concentration of a volatile anesthetic agent. It works by controlling the vaporization of anesthetic agents from liquid form and then accurately controlling the concentration in which these are added to the fresh gas flow.

Work-life balance—a concept including the proper prioritization between work (career and ambition) and lifestyle (health, family, pleasure, and leisure).

Index

Note: Page numbers followed by *b*, *f*, and *t* indicate a box, figure, and table